# And a
# Time
# to Die

# And a Time to Die

THE PAIN
AND LOVE
OF A
JOURNEY
HOME
WITH AIDS

## Frances Bontrager Greaser

HERALD PRESS
Scottdale, Pennsylvania
Waterloo, Ontario

**Library of Congress Cataloging-in-Publication Data**
Greaser, Frances Bontrager, 1921-
    And a time to die / Frances Bontrager Greaser.
      p.  cm.
    ISBN 0-8361-9028-9 (alk. paper)
      1. Greaser, David L., d. 1991—Health. 2. AIDS (Disease)—
Patients—United States—Biography. I. Title.
RC607.A26G6354 1995
362.1'969792'0092—dc20
  [B]                              95-16634
                                        CIP

The paper used in this publication is recycled and meets the mini-
mum requirements of American National Standard for Information Sciences—Permanence of Paper for Printed Library Materials,
ANSI Z39.48-1984.

Grateful acknowledgment is made to Frances and Lawrence
Greaser for photos of David, family, and friends used on the cover
and throughout this book.

Excerpt from "When It Is Over," by Edna St. Vincent Millay is from
*Collected Poems,* Harper Collins. Copyright © 1954, 1982 by Norma
Millay Ellis. Reprinted by permission of Elizabeth Barnett, literary
executor.

All Bible quotations are used by permission, all rights reserved,
and are from *The Holy Bible, New International Version*, copyright
© 1973, 1978, 1984 International Bible Society, Zondervan Bible
Publishers.

To all those parents who
agonize as they watch their child
struggle, hope, despair, and eventually
cede to an untimely death.

And to Lawrence, the co-caregiver,
my strong support, lover, and
primary editor.

# Contents

*Author's Preface* ........................................................ 9
*Prayer for Parents of Persons with AIDS* ........................... 11

1. St. Vincent's Hospital .................................. 17
2. While It Was Yet Dark .................................. 32
3. David .................................................... 48
4. D-Day ................................................... 66
5. What Makes Them Do That? ........................... 75
6. Mother Number Two .................................. 87
7. Living with AIDS ..................................... 95
8. AIDS and the Faith Community ..................... 112
9. Doubts and Faith .................................... 120
10. And a Time to Die .................................. 124
11. Afterword ........................................... 131

*Appendix 1: Caring for a PWA* .......................... 142
*Appendix 2: Uncle David, by Aaron Greaser* ............ 153
*The Author* ............................................. 158

# Author's Preface

All journeys are personal ones. Some are painful. The journey of walking with a loved one who has AIDS is one of plateaus, peaks, and valleys. The road is sometimes tortuous and agonizing. But there is an emotional bonding which is sustaining throughout the pilgrimage. Through it all, a sacred light guides and shines on the path ahead.

This is the story of our journey with our forty-two year-old son David, who was HIV-positive long before we knew it. In 1988 he was critically ill and diagnosed as having AIDS. He died three years later.

We treasure the gifts he gave us—generosity, respect, sensitivity, gratitude, and his continued searching for faith and meaning. We value his showing us the importance of hope. In dying, he taught us how to live. We are grateful that he came to us and allowed us more intimately to touch his life during the dark moments when his life's journey was ending.

We value the blessing of the friendships which upheld us during that early winter of his life. In that upholding they strengthened us. We were not alone.

Dave's story has many heroes. Like the many biblical characters who, though unnamed, made a major contribution in the unfolding of the greatest of all love stories, so David's heroes, though unnamed, have played a significant role in the last phase of his life's journey. God will bless them where we cannot.

*—Frances Greaser*
*Goshen, Indiana*

# Prayer for Parents of Persons with AIDS (PWAs)

Loving God, we intercede for the mothers and fathers and stepparents of persons who have died or are dying of AIDS. We pray for those who gave life and now watch as that life is snatched from them. In these painful and difficult experiences, help them and us to remember that *you do care* and that *your* love is stronger than parent love.

We pray for:

Those parents right now holding the hand of their formerly broad-shouldered son who is lying on a bed of death, body diminished of energy and flesh.

The parents of the beautiful, jubilant daughter who brought so much joy and love to everyone's life, now lying quietly, with hesitant and garbled speech, waiting for death to claim her.

Those parents who are searching for strength and hope in the face of a situation in which they feel weak and helpless. Caress them with your arms of love and infuse them with your strength, as they spend their days caring and their sleepless nights wondering what more they can do.

Those parents who live in places and in circumstances where medical services, medications, and the base essentials for life are absent. Grant them in these dark days of suffering and need a special portion of your love and grace.

Those parents who have recently become aware, or will become aware, that their small child or their adult son or daughter is HIV positive or has AIDS. Dear God, help them in their confusion, denial, and anger not to condemn or reject their loved one—or you. Rather, dear Father, help them to draw close to you and through their love reveal your love.

Grant to those who believe in you the capacity to trust in your never failing grace. For those who do not know you, dear God, grant the awareness of your desire to walk with them through these times of deep pain, doubt, and grief.

For all of us who mourn the loss of loved ones who had so much potential for good, do not allow our grief and loss to keep us from reaching out to those who suffer from this dread disease. Remind us through these experiences of the essential things of life; remind us that life with you can be eternally promising and fulfilling.

Gracious God, help all who walk with their loved ones through the valley and the shadow of death to fear no evil, because you are with them.

May your presence, mercy, and grace be their comfort and sustaining power.

Through Jesus Christ our Lord, Amen.

There is a time for everything
And a season for every
activity under heaven. A
time to be born, and
a time to die.

*Ecclesiastes 3:1-2a*

# And a
# Time
# to Die

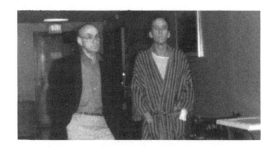

# 1  St. Vincent's Hospital

I stared through the smoke-grimed windows and pondered the rhythms of life. The sun was wrapping New York City in colorful embrace as it drained the sky of its last brilliance. Day was ending in our part of the world, but at the same time, the sun was rising to someone else's pain. Sirens shrieked as police sliced through traffic, yet at a nearby church, bells were tolling the peace that should come at the end of the day. From my vantage point on the seventh floor of St. Vincent's Hospital, over fifty persons were in various stages of dying. Somewhere, just as many were in various stages of being born. God keep them from a similar fate.

Among those fifty dying was our forty-two-year-old son, the son who had boldly insisted that "AIDS was only a virus" and he was going to "lick this thing." Lawrence's son, born in love, and now my son, given in love, was in crisis. We had come to his bedside to help him in his struggle back to health.

This was not an unexpected event. We had first become aware of his diagnosis more than three years earlier when he was hospitalized, seriously ill with histoplasmosis and pneumocystis carinii pneumonia (PCP)—which is almost always associated with AIDS. Since then, we had made few definite plans, except to be available when he needed us. My nursing background and Lawrence's experience in hospital administration gave us insights into the diagnosis. We read books and learned what we could which might help us in this new and frightening experience. Those intervening years were a special gift of making memories together through extended trips, family togetherness, and the unloading of Dave's emotional baggage and concerns. But now the time we dreaded had come.

We had motored from our home in Indiana to Miami, Florida, for a Protestant health convention when the call came from Dave's brother alerting us to his illness. David was too ill to talk to us, but the medical staff whom we frequently called assured us that he was not critical and that they were doing all they could. Both Lawrence and I had responsibilities at the Mennonite health section of the assembly we were attending. Decisions and tensions became unsettling. When we were finally able to talk to David, he insisted that we not interrupt our plans and that he was going to win this battle, just as he had earlier ones.

Our planned trip to Puerto Rico was already canceled. David's illness and the burden of the diagnosis seemed to make other issues trite. We sought counsel from friends who knew New York City better than we, and we left immediately after Lawrence's last meeting.

We were aware that the clothes we brought for Florida and Puerto Rico weather were inadequate for a blustery March in New York, but that was a minor concern.

We left our car at Arlington, Virginia, with my niece and her husband. The next morning they took us to Union Station in Washington, D.C., where we boarded Amtrak for Pennsylvania Station in New York. The aroma and beauty of the budding cherry trees buoyed us, and we would have enjoyed the luxury of indulgence in the season of beauty and new life. Our thoughts were of sadness and death. Yet the promise of new life after a hard winter was what we needed.

The apprehension of the unknown, the suspense of seeing David in his weakened condition, plus the tension of a taxi ride in lower Manhattan produced a vortex of emotions as we unloaded our baggage at a Seafarers Hostel. Now it was time to get acquainted with the noise and confusion of overmotorized New York—a far cry from our placid community in Goshen, Indiana.

The hostel was twelve blocks from the hospital. Although adequate for seamen, I was negatively impressed by the odors, cigarette stubs, and sounds. *Oh, God*, I sighed (most of my prayers began with a sigh). *We believe you want us in New York right now, but is this the place where you want us to stay indefinitely?*

The blustery wind was pitiless as we dodged people and walked south on Fifth Avenue to Twelfth Street, then entered the massive brick structure which housed the physical and emotional sufferers. No one smiled or asked questions as we entered the well-guarded lobby. Everyone knew that a pass to seventh floor meant you were visiting someone on death row. Patients on that floor were not there to prolong life but to prolong dying. Yet after a few days the receptionist began to smile as she automatically handed us our card and said, "David Greaser, Room 781." This bit of familiarity gave warmth and a sense of caring.

It was warmth and caring which had led to David's predicament. David was a registered nurse, blessed with a tender sensitivity. He had been a volunteer in the "Buddy system" and befriended persons with AIDS (PWAs). During his visits with us, he had occasionally told us of the heartache and rejection PWAs feel. He frequently telephoned those people from our house in Indiana, just to cheer them during his absence from them.

Many times he would cry as he finished the conversation. Another person had died, completely rejected by his family, and was cremated the next morning. On one occasion, several years earlier, while David was giving an injection to a PWA, he pricked his finger as he attempted to put the needle back into the container. Now he was hospitalized with active Kaposi's sarcoma. The spots covered his neck, arms, and chest and infiltrated throughout his entire body, especially his lungs.

We walked apprehensively from the elevator. If his dad had not said "Hello, Dave," I would have walked away from the cadaverous mass on the bed, which I did not recognize. His sunken eyes looked like dark marbles in a saucer of milk. His skin was greasy and mottled and hung loosely on his bones. His previously well-managed red hair was receding and lusterless, which made his face look longer.

We knew there was much more, but we saw enough to know that externally and internally, he was being devoured by a monster. The mucus membrane of his mouth was ulcerated from lesions, chemotherapy, and thrush, all complicated by a lack of immunity.

As we tried to absorb the reality, we reached for his hand. David began sobbing, and we tried not to. His mouth was too ulcerated to let him speak. Words were unnecessary but they did help break the stinging silence. We began telling him about our trip, making comments which didn't need an answer.

Finally David, with much emotion, spoke with a weak and slow voice. "I want. . . ." There was a long pause. I moved to the other side of the bed to watch his lips. Then David started again, crying as he forced words to form, "I want to . . . move to Indiana."

We affirmed his decision with much relief and gratitude. Already some of our concerns were gone, but others were just beginning.

The sacred silence of our being together was broken by his roommate, who was simultaneously watching a soap opera blasting on the television and talking loudly and boisterously on the telephone. He made many long-distance telephone calls and seemingly needed to shout his message. David never complained. When I suggested that we consider moving to another room, he said he didn't want to offend Elmo.

Suddenly I became very angry at AIDS. What a murderer! What an infernal waste of human potential! AIDS is shortchanging our society and depriving us of the gifts of thousands who have died and are dying!

I sublimated my anger by rubbing David's washboard back. We talked of trivia. David needed a reprieve from conversations about x-rays, therapy, laboratory reports, complications, and medical directives. We stayed until the end of visiting hours. Did we detect a slightly stronger voice?

We had a lot to think about that evening back at the hostel. From our eighth-floor room, I looked out the sooty windows and listened to the screeching of the cars below. The gray skyline resembled a giant broken-toothed comb, with toy-like yellow cabs darting between the teeth. Little dots of people dodged traffic as they crossed the streets. Only our lives, it seemed, were on hold.

David's condition seemed terminal, yet he wanted to come home. Decisions concerning the length of our stay in New York, where we would stay if we remained, or how to transport David all needed to be faced. David was too weak to leave soon, if ever. What would we do about the car and David's possessions? If he got better and went to his apartment, where would we stay?

Even after one day, we began to fit into a pattern and found a sense of comfort in seeing the same waitress at a restaurant. Renewed by the brisk walk and invigorated by the busyness of the masses, we passed well-known landmarks on the way to St. Vincent's. If we hadn't had heavy hearts, we could have enjoyed New York.

David had had a disturbing night. He seemed to feel a personal responsibility for our comfort in New

York. We had intentionally come to his room at 10:00, which allowed him time for his morning care. He had already showered and had a battery of tests. Both doctors had been there and told him he now had a staphylococcic infection in his back. That explained the lack of closure of a previous surgical procedure.

While returning to New York after a week with us at Thanksgiving 1990, David's plane had hit an air pocket. He developed severe pain in his back but nevertheless toted his big box and luggage to his second-floor apartment. For the next few weeks, he had muscle spasms so severe he could not tolerate going to a doctor.

In early December, x-rays revealed a deteriorated disc. In January, the ensuing surgery with his debilitated condition and its complications had brought him to this spot. It was hard to believe that he had already gained eight pounds since his admission. His eyes had a hint of a glow; he smiled as he saw us come and reached out for the *New York Times*.

After listening to the overnight and morning report, I asked the nurse if there might be a quieter room. In an hour, the nurse came to David and said, "We're going to move you to another room, you will like your new roommate. He's quiet."

David looked at me and grinned, suspecting that someone was already interfering with his life. He smiled knowingly as he slowly put on his red-and-black robe. He leaned on his dad while I guided the IV pole to the last room at the end of the hall.

The new room was a pleasant change and a wee bit of assurance that *something* could be made better. I was overwhelmed by the sight of an entire floor of PWAs, all showing symptoms of their sentences in different ways. Some were coughing, others groaning, some talking loudly and incoherently while others lay still and stared. Kaposi lesions were entangling brain cells, lungs, kidneys, eyes, and legs without mercy. My anger at suffering and loss of potential persisted.

David's new roommate had recently been admitted with severely swollen legs which restricted his employment. His quiet demeanor was healing to all of us. We became absorbed in our reading material. We needed nothing more than just to *be* with Dave, content to sit in silence except for the constant beep of the pump which regulated his TPN (total parenteral nutrition), a nutritious formula which provided his daily sustenance.

A stranger interrupted the silence when he invited us for refreshments in the lounge. Volunteers from St. Luke's-in-the-Fields Episcopal Church provide refreshments for PWAs and their guests every Saturday and Sunday. David encouraged us to go, and we had no reason to refuse. We joined those on wheelchairs, those dragging their IV poles, and those struggling to walk and finding support in their friends.

The conference room, which also served as a lounge, was bare except for two joined formica tables surrounded by plastic-covered straight chairs. Now the room was transformed into a social area replete with carts of luscious rolls, another beverage cart, styrofoam plates and cups, and plastic eating utensils. Volunteers, all men from nearby Catholic, Quaker, and Lutheran churches, joined the Episcopalians in hosting the social hour. They were friendly people and encouraged conversation. Everyone was on a first-name only basis.

It was entertaining enough (if entertainment was what one wanted) to watch those with AIDS shuffle into the room, most of them accompanied by their same-sex friends. One especially attracted my attention, and the verbal banter of the hosts made me guess he had been there a long time. He came in his blue-striped pajamas and enormous lion slippers, accompanied by a woman. The woman's bulging eyes were hidden behind plastic-framed glasses. A coarse, oily complexion and blond, dry hair made me question her identity. The big hands, masculine legs, and flat chest convinced me that "she" was wearing a wig. Comments were few, but when "she" did talk, the voice was deep and guttural. Even "her" body language was masculine.

As we interacted around the table, we inquired about housing facilities nearer to the hospital. A name was suggested. Immediately someone left the table, and soon returned with the address and telephone number. Lawrence contacted the place, but we felt there was no advantage in making the move. This depressed David because he felt a responsibility for our comfort.

Later that same preppy-looking fellow who had gotten us the phone number came to our room and asked what we had decided. He had a broad, friendly smile, with straight dark hair pointing to his right eyebrow. His dark-rimmed glasses could never hide those laughing eyes. Lawrence thanked him for his concern but said we would stay where we are.

His wide grin widened as he handed us a paper with his name, address, and telephone number on it and said, "We'd like you to stay at our house, if you wouldn't mind that we are remodeling. We're seven blocks from the hospital in Greenwich Village and have a second floor we aren't using. It's fully furnished; we keep it for family and friends when they're in the city. You can have it for as long as you need it."

Overwhelmed by the offer, I blurted, "But what are your rates?"

"Nothing!" was his immediate response. "There are some tiles loose in the bathroom, but I will fix them tonight yet. Just call me when you will be there, and I will meet you by the front door." He disappeared as mysteriously as he had come.

Could God's love be made any plainer than that? His providence was being handed to us in ways we could not even imagine. It was an unbelievable gesture of hospitality. We knew nothing about this man, but his demeanor made him endearing and trustworthy.

David grinned, nestled back in his pillow, and said, "Go for it!"

That evening Lawrence called Mr. Arisman and told him we would be there at 10:30 the next morning. We felt akin to Abraham, "walking by faith, not knowing whither we went."

We were entering Holy Week. The next day was Palm Sunday, and worshiping with the Seamen seemed appropriate. We planned to change our residence after the service.

A cross and a palm branch were fixed on the pale

yellow-painted walls of the chapel. The chaplain had a stirring message on the paradox of the agony and the ecstasy of that donkey ride into Jerusalem. We were experiencing our own agony. Would there ever be joy? My timid soprano voice was eclipsed by the lusty voices of the seven navigators who attended the service. The chaplain, we later learned, was no stranger to Mennonites.

Knowing it would be easier to get a taxi there, we carried our bags to Union Square. It was a sleepy Sunday morning with little traffic. The tall buildings dwarfed the streets, making them seem like alleys. The few taxis we saw sped by, either full or on another call.

A station wagon stopped and offered to take us wherever we wanted to go. Another New York surprise! We soon recognized the chaplain with whom we recently had a lengthy conversation. Seeing a familiar face was like a letter from a friend. Were we already experiencing a hint of the joy of that donkey ride to Jerusalem? The chaplain helped put our bags in his car, and we were off to new adventure.

We headed for St. Luke's Place, which has only fifteen houses and is one block long, lined by ginkgo trees which shade brownstone Italianate houses built in the 1850s. Frank Arisman met us and eagerly grabbed our bags, bounded up the eight steps, and introduced us to his blonde, petite wife, Mary Ann.

The front door opened to a tiny area only big enough for boots and a small table used as a mail drop. A second locked door opened to the main foyer with high ceilings and an elegant open stairway leading to another hall and a third locked door which opened to our New York City home. What an oasis amid a desert of monotony and sterility!

Frank delighted in introducing us to our facility. Virgin white walls, two bedrooms, a big living room area separating them, a bathroom, and laundry—all were tastefully decorated in white and blue. An Oriental rug covered most of a white rug on the hardwood floor. There were white tulips on the dresser as well as a flashlight. *From Trout Stream to Bohemia* (Old Warren Road Press, 1988), a history of Greenwich Village by Joyce Gold, welcomed us even more.

The history of Greenwich Village intrigued me. As we looked through the warped windowpanes at the park across the street, Frank told us about the colorful Mayor Jimmy Walker; the park was named for him, and he had lived next door. Previously that park had been a cemetery where Edgar Allen Poe wrote "The Raven." Houses on this short street have been homes to many famous writers, artists, and poets. The artist living on the floor above us has her art displayed at the Metropolitan Museum of Art. Three doors from us, the exterior scenes of the Cosby show were filmed. Some writers have described this as "the most delightful street in all New York City."

Dave's eyes sparkled as we told him about our new facilities. His mouth was still painfully sore, and he rinsed it frequently with an anesthetic solution when he tried to talk. Meals were brought to him routinely and just as routinely carried out—almost untouched. Any effort was exhausting. His skin had a ghastly, translucent purplish appearance. His sunken eyes and loss of fat pads were a grim reminder that death was stalking. Simply sitting beside him required emotional energy, but our gift of presence was healing to him. We silently sat and read.

Frank put a *New York Times* by our bedroom door every morning. We quickly read it, put it at his door, and bought another for Dave. Frank soon informed us that the *Times* was for us and Dave, and he bought another for himself.

Mike Troyer from Connecticut, Dave's cousin, came to see Dave that afternoon. Later his cousin Steve Troyer and Steve's wife, Cathy, who live in New York, both came.

Amid the masses of New York, it was comforting to have family and friends link us with a former life of well-being. That evening we had our first exposure to the Manhattan Mennonite Fellowship. The warmth of that small group compensated for any longings for our home congregation. We belonged immediately.

We were swimming upward in an emotional downstream. The luxury of the whiteness and comforts of our "suite" was a haven during the crisis. After an emotionally draining day at Dave's bedside, it was pure luxury to shower behind Battenburg lace curtains, wrap one's body in extra-thick white cotton towels, and focus thoughts on more pleasant aspects.

Early mornings were ideal for exploring the Battery and other environs in lower Manhattan. We saw "The Lady," Staten and Ellis Islands, and other historical spots from the 107th floor of the World Trade center. We explored Washington Park, absorbed the collegiate atmosphere at New York University, were dwarfed by the mammoth structures along Wall Street, and welcomed the silence of Trinity Church as we meditated there. The intrigue of the area added stimulus to an otherwise draining ordeal. David was always eager to hear about our adventures and had a few suggestions of other nearby places we ought to investigate.

The incision in David's back was continuing to drain. He was quiet and inactive but appreciated our being near him. All the membrane inside his mouth was one big ulcer. Words came slowly. He grimaced and twisted his head when he tried to swallow. We didn't ask him to speak. It hurt him and us. His roommate was blessedly quiet.

David's housemate, Glenn Andersson, came that afternoon. He had dark eyes and hair and an entertaining Brooklyn accent. We had met him before, but he had kept his distance and treated us formally. Discussions centered around finding a spot to park his car and comments about traffic and weather. Lawrence and I walked the corridors of the hospital so they could be alone. It was obvious that Glenn was uncomfortable in our presence.

We knew how much Glenn and his mother and aunt had done for David, and how their home had become his home in Brooklyn. Dave had not excluded Glenn from his conversations with us, yet we observed that Glenn had trouble relaxing with us. His body language revealed that tension. When he was ready to leave, we walked to the elevator with him as we talked.

Glenn's mother, he revealed, was having undiagnosed emotional problems. He could no longer leave her alone in the apartment. His mother's aunt, always the stable one, was now in a nursing home. Glenn, an only child whose father had died in his childhood, was chef at a popular eating place in Long Island. Easter season was especially busy and sometimes he stayed at the restaurant overnight. Now his best friend seemed to be in the final stages of life, and he felt guilty about not being with Dave at home.

The elevator was almost at seventh floor. I looked at Glenn and said, "Glenn, this is really hard on you. You are having a tough time right now. May I give you a hug?"

He looked at me, mystified, then grinned. I stood on my toes and reached up to his shoulders as I encircled his stiff body. Hugging was not in his repertoire of communication. He relaxed and smiled when we said good-bye as the elevator door opened.

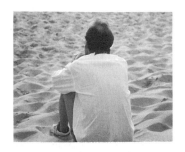

# 2  While It Was Yet Dark

Tommy, an anxious man in his fifties who claimed to be a lawyer, talked incessantly and incoherently. He was restricted in a wheelchair near the nurse's station, where he could be watched more closely. Kaposi's sarcoma lesions in his brain limited his control of his thoughts and comments.

His stories of sexual conquests may have been real or imagined, but they were loud and lewd. We walked by him, deliberately ignoring him to avoid triggering additional comments.

His olive-skinned mother, short, with a body resembling a withered pear, brought him a bag of his favorite food. Her greasy hair fell over a weathered face, and her penetrating dark eyes revealed her anger before she voiced it. But she too needed to be heard. Her anger at Tommy's condition was loudly aired as she wrung her hands and paced the halls, avoiding the laundry bags and supply carts.

"Where is God?" she screamed. "How could he allow something like this to happen to my Tommy?"

"Lady," I said quietly, "God is here watching you suffer just like he watched his son suffer almost 2000 years ago today." This was Good Friday, and the sacredness of the hallowed day sustained us in our own suffering. "He loves and he cares, but we must let him."

"I don't believe it!" she shouted back to me. "There can't be a God. How can any God let this awful thing happen to a good person?"

I could have said that we have choices, and that God doesn't do these things to us, but she was too angry to hear.

"Tommy," she said in a more subdued voice, "was a good boy. He was coming home from work and saw two fellows in a fight. He tried to separate them, but one had a sharp knife, already bloody from stabbing. When Tommy grabbed the knife, he cut himself. Now he has AIDS from the knife! Then his wife left him, and now nobody cares about my Tommy. Where is the justice in that? I don't believe there is a God, and if there is, I hate him!"

That story is only one of the over fifty stories connected to all those PWAs on the seventh floor. Across the hall from Dave was a man from El Salvador with a guttural cough. His mother sat devotedly beside him all day, reciting her rosary while fighting tears and loneliness. Her face had lines like a roadmap, now stained with grief. I inwardly grieved with her and regretted that I could not speak her language fluently.

After two days, the constant straining cough was gone. Life had left the body and already a new person was in his bed. This fellow was loud and boisterous on the phone and to anyone who would listen. He was obviously in the early denial stage of thinking that a blood transfusion was all he needed. Male friends streamed in, bringing gifts and increasing the noise decibels. Hospitals have long ago lost one of their basic intentions of allowing persons to rest.

We talked with Dr. Sheree Starrett, one of Dave's physicians, a specialist in AIDS research, and a sister of Dr. Barbara Starrett, Dave's primary physician. Because of this alliance, Dave was on many experimental drugs which were not yet on the market. David had much faith in his sister-doctor team, which was a great plus in his healing process. As Dr. Starrett left Dave's room, we followed her to the hall. Prognosis and the present condition were important to us.

"His PCP (pneumocystis carinii pneumonia) is localized and improved."

"And his prognosis?"

"It may be as soon as three weeks, or many months. It is unpredictable."

What a death warrant! We thanked her and tried to look composed before we went back into the room. Three weeks! If we were going to honor his request, we had to get him home soon, yet he could not tolerate such a trip.

We began a mental whirlwind of decision making. We wrestled with the gravity of the situation. How would we handle travel arrangements? What would we do with all his possessions? How would we find a doctor in Indiana? So much to do in such a short time! David thought he could be discharged over the weekend. It seemed an impossibility, but if faith would help, we would work with him.

Tears flowed easily when we were away from Dave. Where was the balm in Gilead we needed now? Who comforts the comforter? It was a rough morning for all of us. David had learned that there would be no financial coverage for the very expensive total parenteral nutrition (TPN) he needed if he left the hospital. Since he could not tolerate oral food, the intravenous TPN was extremely important. Other reports were needed before final decisions could be made. There was still some discharge from his back.

In less than a month, we might lose David. If he wanted to move, there were legal issues that needed attention. His dad made comments to alert Dave to the gravity of the situation.

"I said I wanted to go to Indiana, but what is the urgency?"

As tactfully as he could, Lawrence told him that Dr. Starrett said he could be in crisis again in three weeks or maybe longer.

David slumped in his pillow and pulled the covers around him as if to shield his debilitated body from the world. He seemed too discouraged to talk or to care. We hugged him and cried with him. We sat in silence on either side of the bed, each absorbing strength from the other. He needed rest, and we needed a mental cathartic. We walked the blocks around the hospital, but the endless sea of nameless faces did little to revive us. David had not accepted the faith we avowed, and he was facing death. That was our biggest concern.

I wondered about the biblical story of the man who

because of his "importunity" was given food for his children. What was lacking in our prayers? What more could we do?

Before we said good night, as I was rubbing his washboard back, David began to cry. His dad got up and gently massaged his arm. Words were unnecessary. Finally he slumped and spaced his words and energy as he sobbed, "If only I could have faith like you." He sobbed some more.

"You can, Dave, you can," Lawrence said soberly. "It's there. It's a gift. Accept it." But faith and acceptance were too difficult to grasp after eighteen years of living a world away from the devotion he had learned in his youth in Puerto Rico. His only response was "It's too simple."

We prayed with him and left him in God's hands, praying that acceptance would come soon. We were in a quagmire of emotions. How did we simply say "good night," knowing that soon we would say "good-bye"? The special squeezes and "I love you" helped us all.

The night was heavy with the pain of the day. Lawrence began having tightness in his chest, and we worried about a recurring heart problem. The bypass surgery he had had a year before made us sensitive to any chest pain.

We left earlier the next morning, walking amid the acrid exhaust of buses, trucks, and taxis up Seventh Street, across Christopher and Greenwich to Eleventh Street, where St. Vincent's Hospital covers the entire block. David was already showered and in his familiar robe, just as anxious as we that we be there when Dr.

Starrett arrived. David seemed ready to accept the urgency if he heard it directly from her.

When she arrived, David sat up and boldly asked, "What do you mean? Am I going to die in three weeks?"

"What are you saying, what do you mean?"

"They said," and he looked at us, "that you said it might be three weeks."

She stared at us in bewilderment, and we explained to her what we thought we heard her say.

"I said that the Kaposi lesions in the lungs might again appear in three weeks or more," Dr. Starrett replied. "But they can be treated. Or it can be three months; we don't know. But I was only talking about the infection in your lungs, not your life span."

David flopped on his bed, emotionally drained. We apologized. Dr. Starrett smiled in acceptance. We felt the heaviness leave. This was a good reminder for us that when we are anxious, we may not hear the message accurately.

Color returned to David's ruddy face. After that, we had an intensive, therapeutic discussion about plans for next week, how to move David's things, where he wished to be buried, and the disposal of his possessions. His will, life insurance policy, and living will were intact. I realized then how well he controlled his life and what an emotionally strong man he was to be able to discuss the finality of life with such poise.

Fitting the pieces of life's puzzle together does not always make a pretty picture, but the therapy of open communication added an aura of mystery and majesty to life. David, exhausted, relaxed on his bed. When the cleaning lady came in to remove the dirty-linen bag and the red isolation needle container, David smiled at her and asked how her day was going.

David needed to rest. We needed to pull our thoughts together. We tried a new restaurant near the hospital and enjoyed one of the many little parks which dot the metropolis. Pigeons were enjoying the remnants of lunches eaten in the park. Even a cold, concrete park bench is comforting when the mind is boggled. David and we frequently needed space, and this was one of those times.

That evening we accepted Frank's invitation to join him for Maundy Thursday services at his church, St. Luke's-in-the-Fields Episcopal. This was the same church which had originally introduced us to him, for it was through St. Luke's and their relationship with people with AIDS that we met Frank. It is the third oldest church in New York City, built in 1822 and fertile with history. Fire almost destroyed the building in 1981, but people of many faiths immediately contributed money to rebuild this famous landmark. The black wrought-iron fence surrounding the courtyard and tombstones wrap the structure in an aura of reverence.

The candles and soft light set a sacred mood. The majestic sounds from the organ were a balm to an open wound. We sang lustily along with Frank and other worshipers. How reverently amidst pain one hears the words of the cross and discovers new meaning with each reading. The sanctuary was filled, and those in furs and those in T-shirts held hymnals together.

During sharing time, many talked of prayer needs for specific people. Along with a social hour at the hospital for PWAs and their families, the church provides a Saturday evening meal for local people who have AIDS. They have a food pantry and a clothing distribution program.

Frank had earlier told us that about half of the congregation is gay and lesbian. They sat there in shorts and jeans, being blessed by the outflow of love they felt from the congregation. Those usually considered social deviants were being accepted and loved and treated with a respect many of us do not give. I learned that even as one approaches life's seventh decade, attitudes can still be changed. I wondered . . . was St. Paul also referring to these when he said that "There is no difference, bond or free"? I in my piety had kept them bound. But here in a 160-year-old church, those whom their families rejected had found love and acceptance.

After the meditation, appointed members read appropriate Scriptures. We joined the worshipers at the chancel rail and received the elements of the eucharist. Then twelve people from the congregation were asked to come to the dais for foot washing. Twelve buckets and towels were placed on the dais. Those who wished came while the rector draped a towel around himself, stooped, washed their feet, and blessed them. The hurting and the healers of the noisy city blessed us that evening.

Frank intended to stay for the fellowship meal and to read Scripture at the midnight service. We declined and were a few blocks from the church when Frank met up with us. He asked if he and Mary Ann could join us for dinner when Mary Ann came back from Catholic mass. Lawrence told him about the restaurant he had found that afternoon; Lawrence was eager to eat there.

Frank stammered a bit, and said, "It's good food and good service, but it is a front for the Mafia." We thanked him and went back to our favorite dinner restaurant.

The next morning we did something radical. After our usual breakfast at the Hudson Diner just a block from the Hudson River, we decided we were going to smile and say, "Good morning," to everyone we met. Undoubtedly, the intense, hurrying pedestrians would label us as "hicks from the sticks" who were not yet geared to the anonymity of the big city, but this was Good Friday, and there had to be some pleasure somewhere. We wanted to find it.

The results amused us and surprised the recipients. Some passed us without a response, then turned to look at us. Some grinned as they mumbled, "Good morning." Others stared and undoubtedly wondered what planet we were from. One tired-looking lady who was sweeping her steps while trying to keep her cat inside seemed invigorated. She picked up her soft white cat, patted it, smiled broadly, stared, and waved at us as we kept walking. Each wrought-iron fence and gate acted as a guardian to privacy and isolation. No one, it seemed, dared to break that fortress.

David wanted to hear all the details of the previous evening. He became quiet and inactive. He was undoubtedly trying to fit the pieces of his life together while going through his own Gethsemane.

It was a "downer day" for him and for us. His nostrils flared as he gasped for breath. That frightened all of us. His doctor had said his lung lesions were healing; why was he back on oxygen? Were we facing the end before we could take him home with us? Lawrence sat with him in silence. I went back to my refuge in the lounge/conference room where I could be alone and stare at the confusing metropolis below.

I remembered our pastor James Waltner's past Easter message, part of which I had recorded in the notepad in my purse: "Elijah wandered in the wilderness . . . but the angels ministered." Yes, Lord, we sense the presence of your ministering angels, but it is still painful. "It's Friday, but Sunday is coming." There is a promise of a better day. The penetrating pain we are experiencing now will not be permanent. "We are living in a Good Friday world, but we are an Easter people!" I needed that reminder. We are a people of faith and joy and hope. But discouragement comes easily. And it was raining.

We descended in the elevator and followed the hospital employees to the noisy cafeteria. Sandwiches, salads, and fruit were all tightly wrapped, in individual packages. Even the food seemed isolated from contact. We stood in line, listening to the chatter of the employees. In a crowded room, we felt very alone. Did anyone care that we were hurting?

David was resting when we returned, so we explored more of the hospital and found the chapel just as Good Friday Mass was ending. We sat there in silence, grateful for a place of solace. John Rempel, pas-

tor of Manhattan Mennonite Fellowship, came to see
Dave that afternoon. The rain stopped and we went for
a walk. When we returned, David had bounced back to
his optimistic self and inquired about our activity. He
was again in control of his emotions. His physical condition affected our emotions, and we were facing the
Good Friday of our souls.

The next day, David was lethargic but ready to
watch a ball game. I went for a long walk along Fifth
Avenue and watched the pre-Easter bustle. The Mal-
colm Forbes collection of Fabergé eggs and other min-
iatures could fascinate me for hours. David was still
fiercely determined that he was going to get well. We
needed to be ready. The drainage from his incision in
his back was lessening. Tomorrow was Easter. New
life? New faith?

We could accept David's death. It was his lack of
faith which was most difficult. Now, when his mouth
was too ulcerated to talk, did not seem the appropriate
time to push the subject. But would it be too late to talk
about this later? Good Friday. Why is it called "good"?
It was the darkness of the soul, yet it was because of
that darkness that we have eternal light "While it was
yet dark." "Yea, though I walk *through* the valley."
Thank you, God. Joy will come again.

In my journal that evening was a quote from Wil-
liam Sloane Coffin, Jr.

It is so wonderful to know that, despite today's chill and
yesterday's bluster, spring is here. Energy is pouring out of
the ground and into every blade of grass. . . . Likewise, it is
wonderful to know that despite appearances to the contrary,
this is an Easter world.

That Sunday we delighted in new birth, new purpose, unlimited love. Despite the agony of emotional suffering, Easter is the ultimate healer and renewer. Our grief was no more severe than the grief of other parents who were standing by a dying child. God was walking with us and showing us new life as evidenced in the daffodils and crocuses which energized the thumb-nail lawns. Resurrection is victory over suffering. Christ's life did not end on Friday. It is an Easter world!

It was Easter Sunday and the last day of March 1991. Rain and thaw had replaced the snow. The winds were diminishing in deference to the balmy, stimulating breezes of oncoming April. A healing rain had washed away most of the sidewalk debris. The fresh smell of spring in the air invigorated our very beings. We joined others dressed in furs and heels on our way to the First Presbyterian Church between Eleventh and Twelfth streets on Fifth Avenue. That church too was gilded in history. The lilies, the antiphonal choir, and the "Hallelujah Chorus" again reminded us of the victory we can experience. The minister stressed that, despite all the pain, Christ was victorious.

The brilliant morning sun danced through the beautiful stained-glass windows and many lilies perfumed the air; the sanctuary was alive with celebration. *Christ had arisen.*

David had had a comfortable night. Did he seem a bit better today—or were we using different lenses? We relaxed with that observation. Steve (Lawrence's nephew) and his wife Cathy, both attorneys, came to see David that afternoon. David grinned and readily accepted and cuddled the pink fuzzy bunny which Cathy jokingly brought for him.

That evening the Manhattan Mennonite Fellowship was another spiritual oasis in a desert of grief. The richness of worshiping with those of similar faith was refreshing. How delightful to meet friends from long ago amid the anonymity of faceless people. One worshiper was a member from our home congregation.

We celebrated our ecumenicity that weekend. On Maundy Thursday we worshiped with the Episcopalians. We just missed the Catholic Good Friday mass. We celebrated Easter morning with Presbyterians. On Easter evening we met with Mennonites. All worshiped the same God; all celebrated new birth and resurrection. Frank had fresh tulips on the dresser that weekend. We had renewed stimulation. For us it was still dark, but Easter had come.

We wanted to recognize Frank and Mary Ann Arisman's generous hospitality. It buoyed our spirits to be able to come "home" every evening to such whiteness and sanity after an emotionally draining day of tension and distress. But what could a retired Mennonite Board of Missions administrator do for this couple? Frank was director of commodities at the J. P. Morgan Bank on Wall Street and zigzagged across the world in the interests of zinc, gold, platinum. We were fortunate that he was at home during our stay there.

Mary Ann was a lawyer who supervised all the other lawyers of the Coast Guard on Governor's Island. Their 150-year-old house was tastefully furnished. Financially there was nothing we could do for them. Taking them out for dinner seemed one small way of showing our appreciation. Lawyers Steve and Cathy Troyer were included since they could share a commonality with Mary Ann. They were Dave's only family in New York, and we appreciated their frequent contacts with him and the way they had hosted us while we were there.

Frank and Mary Ann, we said, needed to choose the eating place. Frank's spectacled eyes sparkled. "Actually, our favorite eating place is at the end of this street, Anglers & Writers at the corner of St. Luke's and Hudson. Craig, the owner, has two restaurants in one block. At the one he serves drinks. At Anglers & Writers you need to bring your own if you want to drink."

The dinner and conversation was delightful and stimulating. Gregarious Frank entertained us with his account of the opening days of Anglers & Writers, and the long acquaintance he has had with Craig since then. The setting was unusual for hyperactive New York City. Bookshelves lined the walls. Craig had scouted the country for antique furniture. He gathered an assortment of tables and chairs—none matching. Crocheted and handmade lace tablecloths added to the homeyness. There were bone china cups for afternoon tea. Craig encouraged people to come in and read books while they enjoyed gourmet tea or a full meal. Craig's mother, recently widowed, had moved to the city to bake pies for the restaurant. We knew why Frank enjoyed the restaurant, for it had an ambiance of comfort and solitude.

A young man, slim and trim in a plaid shirt and jeans, walked in. Frank called him to our table and introduced us to Craig. We had a lively discussion about antiques and invited him to the antique auctions in quaint Shipshewana, a community near us. We offered to host him if he ever came. He thanked us and left.

The waitress came to take our dessert order. Most of us did not want any. But the waitress said that Craig had given orders that dessert was on the house. Amid our objection and gratitude, we all ordered home-made pie and cappuccino. We expressed our gratitude to our new friend, Craig, and continued eating our pie and coffee.

The waitress was slow in bringing our bill. Finally Lawrence signaled her and asked for the check.

In a noncommittal tone, she said, "There isn't any."

We explained that Craig had given us dessert, but we were paying for the main course.

"No," she insisted. "Craig said there is no bill. It's all on the house!"

We were overwhelmed. Lawrence immediately left and caught up with Craig, who was on his way to the other restaurant. No amount of talking could convince Craig to let us pay.

Frank and Steve stared at each other and agreed that something was going on here. "This doesn't happen in New York City!"

For us, it was a humbling gift of grace from an unexpected source which reminded us that God is with us even in those dark moments of the soul. Between the ashes of Ash Wednesday and the alleluias of Easter is a difficult path of resignation, determination, suffering, and ultimate victory.

Our minister had reminded us in an Easter sermon that when we have "the experience that takes away our need to be in control, then Lent becomes springtime." Perhaps Craig's and Frank's hospitality was one of God's ways of teaching us to receive and give up control. Welcome, spring!

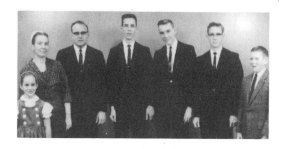

# 3   David

David had entered my life sixteen years earlier when he was twenty-six. He was a robust, brawny, broad-shouldered, handsome redhead, with a complexion as ruddy as the Carolina soil. But sixteen years is not long enough to understand the mystery of the mind. He was always ready to come home for family events but seemed to enjoy them best on the periphery. He brought lavish gifts but did little to initiate any activities.

I had been told that David was "different." David's parents noticed that his interests were different than his sports-minded brothers, but forty years ago the issue of sex-preference was not considered or discussed.

Now we began to silently wonder if he might be homosexual, but we had no proof. When we offered lead comments, he would detour around them. We suspected. But we waited for him to tell us, constantly hoping that we were wrong.

He was an enigma which we tried to solve through conversation and correspondence. He seemed to appreciate letters from us, but he almost never responded. The wall between us had few windows. But the wall came down, brick by brick, when he allowed himself to talk about his sexuality, AIDS, and family implications. The three years after his forced admission of his diagnosis and sexual orientation were a special gift. We began understanding each other. We laughed, struggled, talked intensively, and prayed. Oh, how we prayed!

Three years earlier (1988) David was expected to come home for two reunions for which his dad had major responsibility. It was planned that David would fly to Akron, Ohio, and drive to Goshen with his twin brother, Dan, and his family. This would be a special treat for his nephew and niece. But neither Lawrence nor Dan received any responses to their phone calls. Dave was never home and did not return messages left on his answering machine.

Finally the phone rang. When I heard Lawrence say, "David, *que pasa*? [what's happening]" in a solicitous tone, I immediately picked up another phone. David reported that he had been hospitalized for two weeks because of recurring hepatitis and the opportunistic infection of histoplasmosis. He had a very sore mouth which made speaking almost impossible, but at least he had called. We contacted the hospital and his doctor and learned that he also had PCP (pneumocystis carinii pneumonia) which is almost always associated with AIDS but is not sufficient to diagnose AIDS.

We could only cling to each other and cry, hoping

desperately that our suspicions were wrong. Lawrence wanted to leave immediately for New York, but David insisted that he wait until the reunions were over. Guests were still at the breakfast table the following Monday when Lawrence left to be with David indefinitely.

Seeing a son lying prostrate on a corrugated hypothermia blanket, almost lifeless with extremely high temperature, tubes invading his emaciated body, and machines beeping and whirring is a heart-breaking experience for any father. There were enough signs to convince Lawrence that our suspicions were right. David had AIDS. Everyone on that floor had AIDS. Tears were a bittersweet release for the hurt which father and son experienced. Words are unnecessary when the heart expresses itself. Dazed and brokenhearted, Lawrence sat with his son, trying to absorb reality and wondering why.

Dave struggled to support himself by his elbows and adjusted the tubes in his arms. He forced his mouth to form words. "Dad, I have to tell you that I am gay, and I have AIDS."

His dad could only continue to let the tears flow. He tried to regain his speech. Finally he could say, "Dave, I'm sorry. I am very sorry! But you know that God loves you, and we do too. We will do all we can to help you."

"Whew!" was David's response as he slumped back on his pillow. "What a relief! Maybe now I can finally get some sleep!"

The pain of the diagnosis and the implications of his sexuality stabbed Lawrence as forcibly as any blade could. How did one accept all this? There is no other pain that equals the pain of hearing a son's death warrant. But the next sentence penetrated even more deeply.

"Dad, I just can't believe in God the way you do. I am not sure there is one."

Tears flowed as if a sponge had been squeezed. But the wall was now cracked, and the tears became a fountain of healing relationships. The discussion which followed was the beginning of open communication and shared love.

Lawrence reminded David of something he already knew: "Whenever you are ready or want to, you can come home."

Lawrence stayed at David's bedside for a week—a week of watching him suffer, a week of eagerness for every laboratory report and bit of medical information, a week of despair and an occasional gleam of hope. Our faith in God and daily phone calls were our only consolation. We needed to absorb this reality before we could tell others.

In my need for comfort, I told Dave's uncle and aunt, Weldon and Frances Troyer. Knowing that someone nearby was sharing my grief was a solace. I awaited Lawrence's return, yet wanted him to stay with Dave. Although a stepmother legally, I dropped that title and became a love-mother relationally. How does a mother help a son 700 miles away?

That week of father-son togetherness was a special blessing. They talked of many things: his need to leave his familiar community and move to New York City, the long period of no communication, his reluctance to join freely in family discussions, his homosexuality, childhood experiences, his faith (or lack of it), and his future.

Dave, crying with emotional pain, said, "Dad, from my earliest sexual awareness, I knew that I was different. I tried dating girls in college but didn't enjoy it. I was attracted to males, but I suppressed that."

He wiped his eyes. "I had no choice. It is who I am. It would be much easier to be straight. I didn't choose this. But it's as impossible for me to be straight as it would be for you to be gay. I'd like to be different, but I can't do it."

He felt condemned with no reprieve.

Again his dad felt his muscles tense. "But that doesn't give you liberties to have sexual relationships with a male."

Dave told his dad about meeting Glenn when they both worked at a Fifth Avenue Specialty Furniture Store; Glenn invited Dave to live with him and his mother and great-aunt in Brooklyn Heights, (a different apartment). Dave had become a member of that family and an intimate friend of Glenn. Emotionally drained from the intensity of the conversation, David dropped his head on his pillow. Both were too exhausted to pursue the subject.

David and his four siblings had spent most of their young lives in Puerto Rico, where their parents were missionaries. David told his dad about a fellow in Puerto Rico who apparently was gay, although that term was then unknown. Young people made derogatory comments and gave him many cruel nicknames. David was already aware that he was also different, like Enrique. David had a deep respect for his parents and his nuclear family and knew this exposure would hurt them deeply. The only way to protect them was to let his secret fester within. Like an anchor on a ship, the heaviness of that act pulled him deeper into an abyss.

But when his sexual orientation was complicated by the HIV, he found communication even more difficult. He knew that sometime his family would need to know, but the thought of telling them was excruciating. The wall became higher and thicker. Were not television preachers (and they were the only ones he heard) saying that AIDS was a curse meted out by God?

Rejection, condemnation, and confusion surrounded him. In his youth he had been told of a loving God and was baptized in that love. Why was he being cursed? He sank deeper into his dungeon, fearing that his family might reject him, just as those PWAs with whom he buddied felt complete rejection from their parents. Hearing words of love and acceptance from his father was healing and revitalizing.

David earned a degree in interior design, then added a degree as a registered nurse from New York University. In his responsibility as evening supervisor of utilization review in a large New York hospital, David became aware of many PWAs who were rejected by their families. He watched as their bodies and emotions became more debilitated. The Buddy System, a national organization in which a healthy person relates to a HIV-positive person, appealed to him, and he joined.

When David came home at Christmas, he made

frequent encouraging calls to his dying Buddy friends. He told us about the two lawyer-brothers whose "very religious" parents refused to accept their sons or allow them to come home. Months later we asked about them. Dave hesitantly said, "They both died." There was a long pause. He finished, "They died alone. The next day they were cremated."

David was aware of other similar experiences. Some he talked about them, but most were too painful to discuss. David was already HIV Positive then, but it was too painful for him to tell us. He gave the fateful injection to one of those men. He did it carefully, wearing gloves and understanding the gravity of the situation. As he attempted to put the contaminated needle back into its holder, he jabbed his finger. That instant he became a statistic. That instant changed our lives.

While Lawrence was in New York City, he informed the children of David's diagnosis when he was too ill to attend the reunions, and sent them the following letter.

Dear Galen, Joe and Kristy, Dan and Thelma, Rachel and Steve,

I feel it appropriate to write to you this morning and share some of my struggles, concerns, love, and care for each of you, and something of what has happened during the past week while I was with David, and what I am still trying to cope with. I know that each of you too have your concerns and things to cope with in light of the realities in David's life.

I found it necessary to write down some of my feelings to cope with them more adequately. The enclosed is what I wrote last Saturday alone in my room. As indicated, I told Dave what I had done, and he asked to read it. It had become obvious in our talks that David had been carrying a heavy burden for a long time about his lifestyle and unbelief and not being able to talk about it with us. If on some occasion we (I) had openly confronted him with our concerns and assumptions of how he was living, perhaps we could have gotten through to him. We did try on occasion but, unfortunately, never succeeded.

When he became aware that he had AIDS, it became nearly unbearable for him to tell us. For this reason he didn't tell us about his severe illness which started on June 30, 1988. When he told me the reality of the situation, he said, "Oh, what a relief!" He had been losing sleep for many nights over this as well as his needing to tell us of his rejection of Christianity—knowing that both would be very severe blows to me as well as all the family.

It is probably his agnosticism and his belief that all religions are a myth that is the most difficult for me to cope with. The fact that he was born with genes which, from his earliest awareness, attracted him to men, and his choice of following that drive, undoubtedly also relates to his religious perspectives and decisions. It is not easy to reject and put out of one's conscious and unconscious being the self-condemning temptation of "It's my fault" or to cry out the "why" questions. I know that it is counterproductive and useless to dwell on these kinds of thoughts, and I am trying to overcome them. All I am saying is that it is difficult. I hope none of you ever experience such temptations.

It seems that David has not yet fully accepted the reality of his having AIDS. He frequently says, "Dad, it's only a virus." He said this in the context of reacting to the idea promoted by some evangelists who say AIDS is a punishment from God on homosexuals, and the fear which is so prevalent in our society concerning the disease. Undoubtedly, this is his coping mechanism at work. He does talk about making a will, arranging for possible disability coverage from Social Security, etc.

David was very seriously ill before and when hospitalized. His fever was as high as 106. Glenn's mother spent hours bathing him with alcohol and tried other ways to control his fever. She stuck by him even when he rejected her help because of severe pain and near hallucinations.

Persons who saw him when he came to the hospital, and see him now, remark how much he has improved. It appears that he has been given another chance. His temperature is now below normal and his hepatitis under control. His histoplasmosis will require a long treatment with a medication which can have severe side effects, especially on the kidneys. The fact that AIDS destroys the immune system will, I am afraid, make it more probable that he will have kidney damage.

When David and I talked about informing you of his illness, he asked that I tell you that he promised to write to each of you. I reminded him of our agreement on this matter before I left, and he again said that he would. I noted that he tends to tell friends and family how good things are going, etc., rather than facing reality.

Again, I suppose that is his way of coping. However, he has promised to tell me the whole truth about his condition when we phone him. I tried to impress on him that we can handle the truth easier than handling the suspicion or doubt. He understands that.

We are going ahead with plans to go to Colorado and California in September and October as scheduled with the Mennonite Board of Missions. It is difficult to carry these added concerns and at the same time be a well-primed, enthusiastic conveyer of joy, peace, salvation, and hope in Christ. We are hoping that Dave can spend some time with us in November. He did not want us to cancel any plans. Of course, neither he nor we know if or when he might be able to come for a visit, even if we did cancel plans.

Your cousin Steve Troyer came to see David on Friday. They are good friends. I spent Saturday evening with him. We had dinner together and went to a play in Central Park. He then showed me his office. He is one of 500 lawyers who work for the same company in that building.

I told him about my concern for David's spiritual life, and he told me that he will tell David about his own spiritual journey, and his struggles with issues of faith. Now that I know where David stands on this issue, we can hopefully be in dialogue about these matters in a spirit of love and he will be able to reciprocate in that discussion.

With the letter, Lawrence enclosed the following:

## Issues I Must Cope With

1. How do I relate to David, my son whom I love dearly, in ways that genuinely reflect that love and concern for his physical and spiritual well-being in light of—our prolonged difficulty in communicating openly, including my perception or gut feeling of rejection? This perception was reinforced by the fact that there was *little* reciprocation on David's part to phone calls, letters, etc., as well as being kept in the dark about severe illnesses as he experienced them. In other words, the perceptions and feelings which his mother and I had during the time he worked at Ryder Hospital, and particularly when he left for New York City, that he was "running away,"

have been prolonged by this kind of silence. This may not have been intentional on David's part, but this is how it felt.

On the other hand, there have been a few occasions when we have been together, whether with him in N.Y. or when he came home that were very meaningful and fun, and contradicted the other which I, his mother, and Fran have experienced.

How can this be changed? What can I do, while respecting David's right and freedom as an adult to his perceptions, feelings, and choices, in addition to asking forgiveness for past failures and shortcomings as a father, but at the same time not unduly load myself with guilt and responsibility?

2. How do I cope with the fact that David was born with a homosexual "drive" and has found it acceptable and appropriate as a lifestyle, when my own sexual orientation makes homosexuality seem repugnant and contrary to moral and spiritual well-being for anyone?

Why was David given and born with *this* sexual drive? How do we love and respect each other in the face of this conflicting basic orientation which each of us holds?

3. How do I cope with David's rejection of belief in God, in Jesus as Lord and Savior? How do I handle his belief that Christianity is only a myth, a dogmatic religious idea, alongside other religions? How do I understand and "accept" his doubting or rejection of Christ in light of the fact that our life as a family, including ancestors, has been and is so deeply rooted in faith and in the message of the Bible? How do I release my children, on my gut level, to reject what I feel is so very important for their own present and future well-being? How does God do it and still love, without strings attached?

4. How do I cope with the fact that David has acquired

a life-threatening virus which may subject him to severe illness and an early death? How do I show love, care, and acceptance in the midst of this undeniable reality? How can I be at peace when I know he feels unable to accept the spiritual resources I see as available through Christ for the present physical realities, as well as hope and salvation after death?

5. How can I (we) be present when needed or wanted and absent when not needed or wanted? How can I convey to my family in the midst of these realities that in spite of our failures and sins, God still loves us, still reaches out to us, still offers hope? How can I incarnate that love in the midst of today's realities, in ways that can be freeing, redemptive, and compassionate? I cannot do it alone, but with God's help I commit myself to being this kind of a person, aware that God's grace is sufficient to forgive my past failures and to give strength for today and the future.

Lawrence returned home on August 15. I wrote in my journal:

> Lawrence returned yesterday, ashen and heartbroken. He has lost weight. He is carrying such a heavy burden for his son. His love is genuine, and he cannot stop agonizing. I feel helpless, for I carry the same pain.
>
> My emotions range from sympathy and pity to anger. I am angry at Dave for getting AIDS. It is a deadly disease and he knew that. Why wasn't he more careful? Why didn't he tell us all this when he was with us during the last few years? Why the lack of communication? Why? Why? Why?

Lawrence wrote to his two siblings telling of Dave's

diagnosis and asking their advice about telling their ninety-four-year-old mother. Painful as it would be for us to tell her, we didn't want her to hear it from someone else. Everyone agreed she must be told—by us.

We relied heavily on God's leading as we approached Maple Lawn Homes, a retirement center at Eureka, Illinois. Lawrence told her the story of the injection and said, "Now David has AIDS."

She offered sympathy and love. "Grandma," as she is affectionately known by many, again demonstrated her wholesome, gracious demeanor. Her prayers would be David's and our support during the long struggles ahead of us.

I didn't see David until the following November, when we met him in Chicago at O'Hare International Airport enroute to his cousin's wedding in Hannibal, Missouri. Seeing him so robust, broad-shouldered, and handsome made it hard to believe he had been critically ill three months earlier. I hoped he was right, and that he was "going to lick this thing."

He must have felt the freedom of unconditional love with his family that weekend. Despite his diagnosis, he was hugged and loved by aunts, uncles, siblings, and cousins. He looked and felt great. Dave's twin brother, Dan had asked that David join him at a secluded table for breakfast the next morning. David was usually in slow gear, but that morning the wait seemed excessive. When David finally came, Dan was embarrassed because he had given up and was already eating. There was no apology. David gauged life by his own slow clock. The two of them began their discussion as if time was a nonentity.

That afternoon David told us about the agonizing eternity he had endured that morning when he showered and found the first Kaposi lesions on his arm. He searched further and saw more lesions on his chest. Devastated, he realized he had been sentenced to death. Yet he was determined to fight and win. He had heard of one person who had been in AIDS crisis but had fully recovered and was HIV negative. He would be the second.

The wedding gifts were opened and the festivities ended. We needed to take Grandma back to her apartment in Eureka on our way to Indiana. As we left her there, she reached up to give Dave a farewell embrace. She said, "Dave, I hope to see you in heaven."

David began sobbing as if his heart had broken. To not believe in heaven and hurt his grandma was more than he could bear. We drove on in silence, except for the weeping and sighing in the back seat.

Despite the late hour, there was an intense discussion at our house that night. We prayed that our answers were adequate for his questions.

"If you were raised Buddhist, Muslim, or Jewish, wouldn't you be sure that was the right religion? If you are so sure that your religion is the right one, why aren't you out there converting the whole world? Christians can't agree on a lot of things. Why should I believe any of that confusion?"

God was working. We wanted to be mirrors of his love.

Despite David's diagnosis, those three intervening years were rich, memory-making ones. Especially vivid is the memory of all eighteen family members being together for one week at Joe and Kristy's house in the foothills of the Rockies in 1989. Each day was exciting.

I remember sitting in the lodge at Breckenridge, Colorado, that same week watching the grandchildren ice-skating while the braver grandchildren and adults were skiing. The air was thin and fragile, as if it might break. David developed a fever, headache, and chest pains; I worried about hospitalization so far from home. My anxiety subsided when we realized he was suffering from altitude sickness. His congested lungs could not tolerate the diminished oxygen.

I remember sitting around the stretched-out dining-room table. While the children played with their Christmas treasures, the adults talked seriously of David's condition and our love and readiness to do whatever we could for him.

There are other memories. I remember that special trip the three of us took through Michigan in 1989, and the joy David felt when he could walk through a blueberry marsh and eat fresh blueberries to his heart's content. He felt special pleasure in being inundated by nature's beauty as he sat on a small sand dune along Lake Michigan, just staring at the majesty of the expanse. We had no schedule. He sat there for seemingly hours while we walked the shoreline. We all enjoyed that rough ride on a dune buggy, even when the sand, like small glass pellets, bit our cheeks.

There was the overnight stay in New York City before Lawrence and I left for Israel in 1982, when Glenn hosted us at an exclusive restaurant where he was chef. Later, as we walked the streets of Brooklyn Heights, with David seeming relaxed and pleased that we were there, I asked him why he had come to New York. He immediately replied, "Because I was bored." That seemed a reasonable answer. I needed no further explanation at the time.

In the spring of 1989 we learned to know him even more intimately when he met us at Arlington, Virginia, when Steve and Cathy (whom he called his soul sister) were married.

On another occasion, in 1990, he joined us at Albany, New York, on our return trip from Nova Scotia. We thought we would spend the day with him seeing the sights of Albany, and he would return to New York City that evening.

He had other plans. He came with his bag and was ready to join us in my home community near Buffalo, New York, since he had never been to Niagara Falls. We were happy to go there again. It seemed important to pack a lifetime of experiences into a few concentrated years.

The drizzling rain did not deter us from having a delightful trip in our camper as we sought back roads through the Catskill Mountains and enjoyed magnificent fall foliage. He showed us the house he and Glenn planned to buy. We never did find that perfect spot for a cup of tea on a damp afternoon, so we made our own. With water heated in our camper, we stopped along the soggy roadside and sipped tea from mugs as the raindrops made magic designs on the windows and our in hearts. The coziness of the camper and the warm tea cemented a magical bonding.

The next day he had more opportunity to become mesmerized by water as he contemplated Niagara

Falls. He disappeared. We became concerned, until we found him behind scrubby bushes staring at the water *before* it plunged over the cliff. I wondered if he was pondering the analogy of his life, but words were unimportant. When one is invigorated by God's majesty, words sometimes interfere with worship.

Dave enjoyed another family reunion that following summer 1990 and spent two weeks with us in November. During that time he commented, "Statistically, a person with HIV lives three years after the first opportunistic infection. I am going into my third year. That's scary!"

During his trips home, Dave became acquainted with our minister, listened to the tape of sermon on AIDS Pastor Waltner had preached, read the AIDS packet from Mennonite Mutual Aid, and was pleased with all he read and heard. We compared books and he suggested more. We shared a mutual understanding of the problem. We were in it together.

On Thanksgiving Day we celebrated both Christmas and Thanksgiving. As usual, he left with an enormous box filled with artifacts for his friends, for the apartment, and for Glenn and his mother. Glenn's mother was becoming increasingly disoriented and beginning to hallucinate because of her emotional problems. This was disconcerting for Dave, for she was his New York surrogate mother.

On the return flight from Indiana, David felt a severe jab in his lower back when the plane hit an air pocket. Despite the intense pain during the remainder of the flight, he took a subway and a taxi to Brooklyn with his garment bag and big box in tow. He climbed the flight of stairs and collapsed in his room. The muscle cramps were too severe to allow him to taxi across town to see his doctor. He waited a few days, but the pain did not lessen.

David's days were long and painful and we were entering the Christmas season. Glenn was busy as a chef and often needed to stay near his restaurant overnight. David lay in pain with no one to care for him except Glenn's disoriented mother.

Long-distance phone calls were inadequate caregivers, but communication was open. We encouraged him to go to a hospital. He thought he would be better when the muscle spasms stopped. After what seemed an excessively long time, he was able to ride the subway and taxi to his doctor. In January 1991, he was admitted to a hospital and surgically treated for a deteriorated disc. Soon after he was discharged. He was put on disability pension and said he was going to do all the things he had wanted to do but couldn't because of employment. He resumed intensive treatment for AIDS, followed by severe side-effects.

The following March 1991, when we were unaware of the complications, he was again admitted to the hospital, severely debilitated. The condition of his T cells and hemoglobin was almost incompatible with life. He knew we were going to a health convention in Florida and did not want to spoil our trip. He had been hospitalized for over a week before he allowed Glenn to reach us through Galen in Texas.

That was the phone call which brought us back to New York and to what we thought would be the end of David's earthly life.

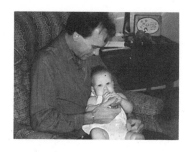

# 4    D-Day

The cultural and historical aura of the formerly Bohemian New York added stimulation to our daily hike to and from St. Vincent's. David, by contrast, had little but bare walls; red plastic isolation bags; a smoke-grimed window overlooking an unkempt, cluttered courtyard; and a will to leave all this imprisonment.

These were busy days at the hospital. We had been with Dave over a week and already the word *discharge* seemed to make David hopeful, although we were more doubtful. He was forcing himself to eat, and the walks through the hospital halls with his father were becoming longer every day. A neurologist had checked him and ordered another medication. The incision in his back was healing. We had a doctor available if and when Dave arrived in Goshen.

Dr. Starrett was ready to write the liberating word when it was discovered that some of the insurance forms were not properly filed. Disappointment was no stranger to us. Dave began chilling and nestled back under his sheet. He needed rest.

We walked to Sixth Avenue to get copies of Dave's medical records at Dr. Starrett's office. Again we were distressed by the damage done by AIDS. Nine young men were draped over the stuffed chairs in the waiting room, most of them pale and sallow-skinned, grasping for life but expecting death as fluid dripped into their veins. Nurses stepped over legs as they monitored IVs and vital signs.

Those professional people who daily nurture the suffering and dying—while trying to make their final experiences in life more bearable and satisfying—deserve accolades. In November 1993, the Center for Disease Control (Atlanta, Ga.) reported that approximately one million people were infected with AIDS just in the United States, representing approximately one in 250 Americans. From July 1992 to June 1993, 315,390 cases of AIDS and 194,344 deaths were reported. When will this tragedy end?

As we left St. Vincent's Hospital, the sun was trying hard to push its way between the rows of buildings, chased by dark, damp shadows. We were becoming more adept at pedestrian patterns based on ignoring street lights but listening to taxi horns. We dodged same-sex couples and hurrying people as we zigzagged on the crowded sidewalks, illuminated by the glitzy neon signs of the storefronts. New York is busy all day, but at night it becomes alive.

The flurry of last-minute activities bombarded us, but Frank and Mary Ann wanted to take us to dinner at one of Frank's favorite eating places—a renovated warehouse along the Hudson River. Each table was isolated in a small, secluded nook where writers and poets could contemplate their muses while they ate. Apparently creative juices flowed more freely in that atmosphere. Did anyone, I wondered, author a book on AIDS in that setting?

Frank, we had noticed, did not drink alcohol nor smoke. We smiled as he ordered a glass of iced tea and three glasses of ice cubes. His conversation was always stimulating and his encounters entertaining. Lawrence asked him what he enjoyed most. "Frankly," he said, "I get my kicks out of going to church."

The conversation centered on his experience as a lay leader at St. Luke's-in-the-Fields and his former church near State College, Pa. How serendipitous it was for us to have met Frank among the millions in New York City. But serendipity and coincidence were not in our vocabulary. We were dealing in miracles, and we had them almost daily.

Finally Dr. Starrett was ready to write the words "Discharged in the a.m.," and David began anticipating the magic air of freedom. Tomorrow would be D-Day. We had the bag of medications intact, and a doctor and other resources were available to us in Goshen. We felt ready to tackle the next adventure.

Lawrence and I had planned that one of us would ride Amtrak to Washington, D.C. We wanted to get the car we had left with relatives in Arlington, Va., and take it to David's apartment in Brooklyn. We knew that David was too weak for that extra trip to Washington D.C. When he learned of our plans, he insisted that he go with us on the train.

We weren't ready to grant his wish but were becoming more aware that David had internal fortitude few of us knew. David, strong in his vulnerability, yet mellowed by weakness, began to mentally vacate his apartment. Steve stopped in to say farewell to his cousin. Both spoke with a bravado which shielded the pain of their last conversation.

"I couldn't sleep until 3 a.m.!" David told us the next morning as he came toward us in shirt and trousers—trousers which hung on him like pants on a clothesline. He had found a bathtub and was refreshed by a therapeutic soaking. His gaunt appearance was overshadowed by a determined expression of victory. He was going HOME!

Twelve days before we had seen him pitifully emaciated and listless. Now he was *walking* out of the hospital. He refused a wheelchair, walked to the elevator and pushed the button. He was again in control of his life. He squared his shoulders as he walked through the massive lobby toward the front door and the dazzling sunlight. Deprived of fresh air for a month, even the unswept streets, cluttered by windblown papers, blinking signs, and hyperactive people, looked inviting to him.

Lawrence hailed a taxi, and David stared out the window as we started our thirty-minute drive across the Brooklyn Bridge to his second-floor apartment on Forty-third Street in Brooklyn. Seemingly empowered by unknown strength, he walked up the flight of stairs. The disoriented Mrs. Andersson opened the door.

David made a quick tour of the small two-bedroom apartment, rearranged things to his taste, and said to me, "I can't believe how much Juana has changed. She walks and stares like a zombie."

Mrs. Andersson had said to me, "David looks so bad. I never saw him look this bad before. I am *so* sorry!"

There was no time to rest. David had earlier arranged that a co-worker would bring boxes for packing. I searched the cupboards for items to make a nourishing meal, for my responsibilities began when we left the hospital. I needed to find food which was not only nourishing, but palatable, soft, bland, and high in carbohydrates and calories. Glenn was exceptionally busy at the restaurant and would not be home. A home-cooked meal seemed to invigorate Dave. We were pleased to see him eat so well.

The doorbell and telephone kept ringing, and friends poured in to celebrate his homecoming and his homegoing. David worked with and supervised fellows from Turkey, Haiti, Puerto Rico, and India. It was a cosmopolitan evening with lots of conversation and laughter.

We stayed in the background so David could be alone with his friends in the crowded room. Most came to the kitchen to tell us how much they enjoyed working with him and of his genuine personal interest in each one's problems and concerns. It was obvious that he was not only their supervisor but also their friend.

David was torn between wanting pleasantries with his friends and getting on with the job of decision making. He ignored our strong appeals to relax. But after his friends left, his defenses failed him. He began to chill, groan, and cry uncontrollably. We sat by quietly, rubbing him gently, avoiding the purple lesions on his forearm and behind his ear. His clothes were damp from the perspiration. His facade was slashed by lack of sleep and the tensions of the day.

But within ten minutes he grinned, said, "Thanks, I'm in control now," and was ready for more food. His dad had already walked to the nearest grocery and bought him the Häagen-Dazs ice cream he craved.

We taxied to our Manhattan "suite," invigorated by the New York skyline at night. The next morning we celebrated David's homegoing by walking to the battery and across the Brooklyn Bridge, taking a taxi from there.

David and Glenn had talked into the early morning. Friends of eighteen years were being physically separated. David said later that Glenn awoke often during the night and realized that he was crying. Glenn was gradually realizing that his bravado does not cover his need for friends and family. The loss of David and the worrisome debilitation of his mother was also weakening him.

Dave had made lists of things to be sent to Indiana. We followed him from closet to cupboard to drawer, taking possessions as he pointed to them, packing and labeling the boxes. Eleven boxes of clothes, heirlooms, and other valued objects were taken to the United Parcel Service office.

The day was one of organized confusion, disjointed by phone calls and visits from Home Health Care and social workers who needed to be sure that Dave would receive continued care in Indiana. There were address changes and services to discontinue. Dave's

Haitian friend, Gene, was there with his car for all errands and eventually to take us back to St. Luke's at night. The next day would be V-day, and we were beginning to believe it might happen.

It was planned that we would meet David at a specific taxi area at the Penn Terminal on the lower level of Madison Square Gardens. We arrived and waited and waited. Tension mounted. Was David too sick to travel and had no way of notifying us? Or was he just moving exceptionally slowly this morning? We stationed ourselves at two spots, hoping we had visual coverage. But finding someone in that hubbub of moving humanity seemed impossible.

Finally Lawrence remained as sentinel, and I went down to the main terminal where pedestrians, like ants, were scurrying. My eyes scanned the masses, but it appeared hopeless. I checked the benches to see if he might have collapsed. At last amidst the raucous noise I heard David call my name. Glenn had in desperation parked illegally near a different taxi station and could not leave the car. Dave had come with his backpack, garment bag, and medicine case and miraculously found me in the crowd.

It was another miracle, but we were becoming accustomed to them. We made our connection, and the porter graciously arranged space for us to be together enroute to Arlington, Va.

During the night in a motel enroute to Indiana, the moon peeked teasingly through the draperies of our room. I awakened to see David staring in front of the open window, seemingly unmindful of the cold spring air blowing over his almost nude body. For a moment I could only allow myself to imagine what was going on in a mind so full of pain, adjustment, and separation-anxiety. Such a quick move from the deafening noise of the big city into the sereneness of a pastoral country setting must have been overwhelming.

I tried to empathize with what he was experiencing, but my motherly admonition took over. "David, you've got to put some clothes on or wrap in a blanket if you are going to stand by that cold air." He took a blanket and continued standing there. Eventually he went to bed—but probably not to sleep. We ached with him and wondered if it was wise to move on.

He was up early the next morning, had a healthful bowl of oatmeal, and went outside while we gathered the baggage. We saw him leaning against the car, staring at the sunrise as he absorbed the beauty of nature. His eyes followed the flight of a robin as he listened to its song. As we approached, he looked at us and said, "It's great to be alive!" and folded himself into the front seat of the car.

I nestled myself in a corner of the backseat, so he could fully recline and relax as we drove westward. That plan was quickly nixed. He sat upright, not wanting to miss any of spring's brilliance.

We began wondering if we should drive directly to Goshen with our precious cargo, rather than stopping at son Daniel's home near Akron, Ohio, as planned. By late afternoon, David was getting exhausted.

We took our weary passenger to Dan and Thelma's home, where he could relax overnight. Their children, Aaron (sixteen) and Danita (eleven), were awed by his appearance. The Uncle Dave they remembered was a robust, smiling person interested in whatever interested them. This was not that uncle. Dave took his pills, ate some noodle soup, and went to bed. He was anxious to have the trip end. So were we.

He had a fitful night. We left the house at 10:30 the next morning, on April 8, 1991, David was happy to relax in the reclining seat but remained fascinated by the open spaces of the country, the smells of the newly plowed fields, and the sounds of the bird songs. The beauty kept him from sleeping.

All of us became more attentive as we neared Goshen. He was going to make it! As we drove in our driveway, we immediately opened the front door so he could come in and collapse on the davenport. He had other business. Before he went inside, he walked around the house in his stocking feet to see if the tulip bulbs he has planted last fall were coming up. He grinned as he came in saying, "They made it!" Then he relaxed.

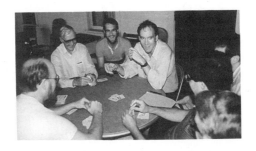

# 5  What Makes Them Do That?

"And so, David is with us. We don't know if it will be for a month, three months, six months, or a year—but we will take care of him until he dies."

We had just finished telling our Sunday school class of over 100 about our experiences of the past month. We had no qualms. They were our church family, and tragedy among us need not be borne alone. We knew there would be support among God's people, for pain draws the people of God together. Some might be judgmental, but that was their prerogative. It is always easier to be critical when you have not experienced the pain.

But we had not anticipated the overwhelming support we felt after the service. Their tears mingled with ours as we were hugged and loved into a warmth of caring far beyond our expectations. At that instant we knew that we would be empowered for whatever lay ahead. There was more healing in the corporate worship which followed. We had missed our church family and were renewed by handshakes, exhilarating singing, and the heartening message.

David was listless when we returned. We had been back in Goshen for a week. Our forty-two-year-old independent and self-directed man had become a child again. He welcomed my arms around him as he struggled to master the pain of living. But soon he was again in control and suggested that we go for a ride after lunch.

David's stamina was as unpredictable as the weather we were experiencing, but a ride through the backroads of Indiana led to surprisingly beautiful pastoral scenes. The beauty of the early spring flowers pushing through the decayed leaves refreshed us, even as it aerated our minds. Why was I suddenly seeing so many birth-death-birth analogies? April is a rejuvenating month, full of surprises. It is a capricious gift of elaborate splashes of friendly and warm colors, sudden earth-awakening rains, threats of violent tornadoes, and assurance of balmy days. So much of our life was becoming like April.

The extra bedroom on the main floor had been transformed from my study/sewing room to a bachelor pad befitting David's taste. He had had his introductory visit with Dr. Frechen, who would be his primary physician. There were phone calls to Dr. Starrett's office in New York to provide adequate follow-through. Oxygen and its ominous machine were part of our house furnishings, and a fifty-foot telephone cord allowed Dave the privacy and convenience of energy-saving phone calls.

David's face lit up when he met Joyce Bontrager,

the Elkhart County AIDS education nurse, for they had been classmates at Hesston (Kan.) College. She came often, supplied him with books and information on community resources, answered questions, and arranged for him to attend a support group in South Bend, a city thirty miles away.

David seemed content in his new environment. And when discouragement hit, his sister, Rachel, would come with a new perspective, bringing food, flowers, suggestions, enthusiasm, and especially her three children. They furnished the laughter and antics he needed. Meal planning continued to be a problem, but the satisfaction of having him home compensated for any stress.

Our small world seemed smothered by a deathly cloud, but we soon learned we were not alone. The doorbell rang, and a friend was there with warm, freshly baked sweet rolls. David enjoyed them so much that she was asked to bring more. She soon became known as "the sweet roll lady."

That was the beginning of an outpouring of love's gifts from so many friends. Their offerings in the midst of our pain renewed our assurance of God's caring. It also exercised our need for humility in accepting this generous caring. Never had we felt so buoyed and sustained by the knowledge of that incomprehensible gift of prayer.

David's image of "midwest conservatism" was quickly shattered when his dentist repaired the tooth which broke while he was eating soft foods. Dr. B. accepted him the same day we called. While putting on his mask and gloves he said, "David, this is to protect you from whatever infection I might give you. I am more dangerous to you than you to me." Dave came home saying, "He was the best dentist I ever had. I felt no pain."

One of our church's small groups became aware that David was missing news from his home community. The next day we were informed that the *New York Times* would be arriving daily at their expense for as long as David was with us. When David learned that, he looked at Lawrence incredulously and asked "What makes them do that?" It was one more opportunity to tell him that caring begins with a God who cares. God's people heard of a need and acted on it. David labored for an entire day over his thank-you note for that superb gift. He was experiencing God's family in ways which were shattering his former concept of an absent or silent God.

Another friend who had previously brought deboned chicken and jellied broth rang the doorbell and waved as she drove out the driveway. Stuck in the screen door was a personalized prayer for the day.

During the second week of Dave's stay with us, all his siblings came home—from Ohio, Texas, Colorado, and Indiana. David had received two units of packed red cells but was still feeling miserable. Although stimulated by being with the family, he spent most of the afternoon in bed, undoubtedly torn between the joy of seeing them and the agony of knowing why they had come.

We had told very few that the children were coming, but the news had spread and food appeared. A friend came apologetically with a large platter of cookies saying, "I hadn't heard about your hurt, and I am sorry I didn't come sooner, but when children come home, they need cookies." The "sweet roll lady" came through again, and David proudly showed off the rolls his friend had made.

I heard him tell his siblings how overwhelming all the food, cards, telephone calls, and visits were. He didn't mention prayers, but I noticed that when someone mentioned praying for him, he looked appreciative.

During the family's stay, the siblings visited local nurseries. David chose a flowering plum tree which was dubbed "The Greaser Tree" and planted on Rachel's property. Everyone knew why it was being planted. With death, there must be visual reminders of life and comfort and beauty.

Staring daily at the face of death eventually sapped our energy and left us discouraged and sometimes critical. Such feelings were alleviated whenever a friend suggested we have lunch. I have many friends to thank for that gift.

Equally important to us were two other couples who would invite us to meet them at a restaurant late in the evening for a cup of coffee and fellowship. Those breaks were a refreshing time of laughter and ventilation of the mind. Laughter was in short supply, and we needed all we could find. The greater gift was that they knew it was important for us to get away and talk of something other than medical appointments or diminished oxygen supply.

A cousin who had a cabin by a nearby lake gave us a key and an open invitation to use it whenever we wanted. Our octogenarian neighbors, who were facing the concluding chapters of productive lives, frequently asked what they could do to help. They kept us supplied with plastic shopping bags which lined all the wastebaskets.

When David was suffering from a severely sore mouth which no medication seemed to help, a friend (who was herself walking through the dismal valley of uncertainty caused by cancer) suggested a mouth rinse which helped her after her chemotherapy. Neither Dr. Frechen nor his nurse had ever heard of the medication but they called all the local pharmacies until they located it.

That friend continued her personal interest in David's welfare. When she called to ask about David, I sensed deep empathy rooted in her own suffering. She gave us the valued gift of realizing that personal pain makes one more sensitive to the pain of others.

Loving is more than a service, for it is shown in the attitude in which it is given. Once a caring couple David had learned to love stopped in just long enough to show him the clever plaque they had made for their grandson. His grin told us that he felt accepted by those a generation older than he.

David's grandmother, who had moved to the community a few years previously, was important to David (and to all of us). On his better days, he enjoyed spending long hours with her, listening and learning. After such a visit he commented, "When I am around Grandma, then I have to believe there is a God." Experiencing her saintly concern had once been encouraging. Now it was sacred.

Our moods rose or dropped like a barometer, depending on David's stamina. The regular flow of greeting cards for him and for us was a constant reminder that others were easing the load. The ingenuity of those who showed their concern was sometimes surprising. In a world of confusion and anxiety, it was good to know that there was a world of order, stability and so much love. Of all the gifts we received, the greatest was that David was accepted as a person of worth, loved by God and by so many others. Friends saw beyond the skin lesions, the pasty skin, and thinning body to the heart of one of God's children.

When we thought everything was going well, David got a cold, which upset us greatly. This was his first cold in three years. What else could we have done or not done? David had a chest x-ray. The bloodwork, though not normal, was satisfactory. He was on antibiotics. We would once more ride the emotional seesaw. He was passive, but in no extreme pain.

Trennis and Elizabeth suggested that we accompany them to see the dogwoods in bloom at her sister's home nestled among the hills in lower Michigan. For David and for us, the beauty surrounding us in that setting was a worshipful experience, even though he had almost no energy to walk. We kept the car windows open on the way home so he could get more oxygen. Yet he gratefully insisted that the beauty was worth the pain.

The telephone was ringing when we came home. Dr. Frechen told us that further checking of David's tests had revealed that he had PCP (pneumocystis carinii pneumonia) in both lungs and needed to be hospitalized immediately. David insisted that he not be hospitalized. He already had a Medi-port inserted in his upper chest which allowed him to give himself his own intravenous medications. Dr. Frechen consented and ordered the appropriate medications from CareMark, a medical supply center in Fort Wayne, fifty miles away. David was allowed to monitor and give his own medications. My anxiety abated. PCP was at least treatable.

CareMark came that same afternoon, bringing the IV fluids, pole, medications, and all other needed supplies. I had a degree in nursing, and Lawrence was a former hospital administrator and his first wife died of cancer. We both knew about illness and death. But David was forty-two and too young to die. This was happening too soon!

I was already too emotionally involved. When Elizabeth stopped with some luscious sweet cherries, she asked how he was. With tears, I said, "I need a shoulder to cry on."

She gave me her shoulder, reinforced by a hug. When a child of God suffers, another child of God responds. And then there was dear Mona (not her name). How good to have time-out with her! Our discussions were deep and serious, for she had a homosexual son living in San Francisco and was fearful that some day she would get a phone call similar to ours. Our admission of David's homosexuality opened the doors for many to come to us with concerns about their homosexual sons or daughters.

We were pleased when Barbara included David in an invitation to a meal at her house. Anticipation is part of the pleasure of any event, and the invitation sustained him through the week. Sadly, when the day arrived, David was too ill to go but insisted that we go.

Disappointment was no stranger to us. This unpredictability kept us from making any permanent plans. Dr. K., a personal friend, wanted to get acquainted with Dave and discuss many of the issues with which Dave was dealing. But David never knew when his mouth would allow him to talk. When he was ready, Dr. K. had other commitments or was out of town. David never got his pontoon ride on the lake for that same reason. When we wanted to schedule an occasion he asked, "How do I know how I am going to feel by then?" Schedules were exchanged for spontaneity.

We did enjoy a scheduled evening of watching David's Uncle Weldon and Aunt Frances embark on a hot-air balloon ride. We followed its flight until it landed in an open field an hour later and brought them back to Goshen. Those two were especially significant in David's experience with us. They had visited him in New York, and had developed a relaxed camaraderie with him. Fran came frequently with food, ordered flowers sent to him, and when appropriate, engaged him in stimulating conversation.

David's Uncle Dana and Aunt Verna were just as faithful with visits and food they knew Dave would enjoy. Verna excelled in making curry and seemed to know when David's mouth was healed enough for him to enjoy it. Dana, recently retired from his opthamology practice, came often and told stories of India, where he and Dave's mother had lived with their missionary parents.

When Dave's Aunt Frances learned of his enjoyment of classical music, she suggested that he come to listen while she practiced on the organ for our Sunday worship service. We sat in the empty sanctuary while she played in the balcony. David was entranced, then hesitantly suggested that we go to the balcony to watch the pedal movement. He clung to the railing while he pulled himself up the steps. His physical pain was overshadowed by the awesome intricacies of that celestial music.

A distant friend, whom I had previously known only professionally, began sending regular notes. She wished we could "spend time together over a cup of tea." Since we could not do that, she sent me a tea bag so we could enjoy the moments in absentia.

Lawrence came home from a meeting and brought a gift from a friend—a football chrysanthemum decorated with a smiley-face made from pipe cleaners. David needed laughter and smiles, and our friend Bob knew how to make smiles happen.

A friend invited me to accompany her to a distant city to attend the funeral of the mother of a mutual friend. I reluctantly refused because I felt needed at home. When Lawrence heard that, he insisted that I go. "Why not? He's not going to die today." I enjoyed an entire day of companionship, an oasis of freedom, with two special friends.

A friend who lived some distance away gave the special gift of herself. Ann arranged for the two of us to spend the day together in another area, which gave me complete freedom to enjoy her friendship apart from concerns for David. Our acquaintance began thirty years ago but when we see each other, we can begin our conversation where it ended the last time. Ann's gift of friendship and memories is precious.

After six weeks at home, friends continued to push out the periphery of our condensed world. In the midst of the dark night of the soul, there were always glimpses of light. In a time of discouragement, worry, and seemingly helplessness, a friend came with brownies, grinning as she apologetically said "These are just for David." She knew Lawrence's diet did not permit them. "Amazing!" David exclaimed, as the goodies rolled in.

Whenever he was hospitalized to receive platelets, the nurses were usually cooperative and friendly. But one evening when David was ready to have his IV discontinued, a pious-looking nurse walked in, gowned and gloved. She cleansed the area and carefully withdrew the needle. She used blameless technique but never said a word to any of us during the procedure. We could only smile and say, "She has a problem." Her body language told us that she was uncomfortable with what she was doing.

A minister friend David had known from his youth came to see him. After the initial free-flowing conversation, the minister looked seriously at him and said, "How does it feel to come home to die?" How would *anyone* answer such a question? David enjoyed it most when others initiated the conversation with stories and experiences, then encouraged his comments.

It is impossible to review the experience of having David with us without remembering all the gifts of caring. To personal friends who gave of themselves so generously, we owe unlimited gratitude. Their name is legion; knowing we cannot name them all, we have named few. God knows who you are and is blessing you for your loving support.

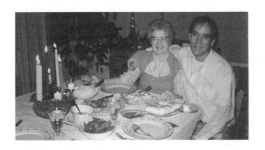

# 6 Mother Number Two

"And how is Lawrence's son?" they asked. It was a kind, well-meaning question, but whenever I heard it, I wanted to say "You mean *our* son?"

They didn't know the heart pang such a question can give, for there is more than one way to be a mother. David was born of love to his biological parents, but he was also given to me in love. I claimed him. He was mine. Although I didn't physically feel the developmental changes of the fetus, or bring him to birth, or observe his childhood development, he was still my son. And now he needed me. Giving birth is not necessary or sufficient for mothering happily or well.

David was long into adulthood when I met him the day before I married his father. I missed a fundamental part of understanding him. That is my loss, and I accept that. After his biological mother died, his father and I acquired a new love between us. We affirmed the sharing of our resources, which included Lawrence's delightful family of five.

I joyfully accepted my new family, which included Galen, Daniel and David (twins), Joe, and Rachel. I, who had never mothered a family of my own, was wedded and welded to this family of four noisy brothers and one sister; they had spent most of their childhood in Puerto Rico.

When I first came into the family, Dan and Thelma were the parents of baby Aaron, our only grandchild. Now we have eight. The grandchildren and their parents soon became main characters in my autobiography.

I enjoy all the children, but it is an adult relationship. I cannot ask or expect them to consider me their mother. But those of us who have never borne children, either by choice or circumstance, can still perform motherly acts. Most women know how to be supportive, nurturing, sensitive, and communicative. These are traits not acquired while giving birth.

I still cringe when referred to as stepmother. The word is born of loss and often carries a negative connotation. That stereotype is being diluted today, for there are over 1,300 new stepfamilies formed daily.

I am reassured when I remember that God *chose* a stepfather for *his* Son. The Nazareth townfolk referred to Jesus as "the carpenter's son"—never as his stepson. Joseph modeled positive stepparenting. His was not a dysfunctional family. A second mother can provide a comfortable home to which children can return and witness their father's return to happiness. At this stage, being a friend is more important than claiming the title "mother."

My grandchildren have never known another

grandmother. When first grandchild, Aaron, was old enough to comprehend the death of his biological grandmother, he said, "I don't care! *She* is my grandmother now!" I enjoy grandmothering.

On Mother's Day I receive the symbols of love from the children—flowers, cards, gifts, or phone calls. I treasure them all. David, extremely generous with Christmas gifts, took little initiative in making contacts during the year. We usually initiated the phone calls, which included a bit of teasing about his negligence in calling us. We could sense the grin as he'd say, "I know I should, but . . ."

After David and his dad had their in-depth conversation at the hospital, the cards and phone calls came more frequently. On his last Mother's Day with us, he and Lawrence bought me a magnificent white rose tree which bloomed profusely all summer. It was planted in the patio near the door, where we could constantly enjoy it.

Apparently the rose tree was not enough. By mid-May I was overwhelmed by the exhausting routine of thinking of five daily meals of adequate nutrition and variety plus our own low-cholesterol needs. The heavy clouds obscured the sun, and the atmosphere seemed to dampen my ability to cope. Self-pity weakened me. I began thinking how nice it would be to go out for dinner on the day that honors mothers—even step-mothers.

David was too weak to let us consider that. There was no choice, so I continued mashing the potatoes, grateful he was still with us. I loved David as I believed I would have loved my biological son. How could one do less? Each child needs specific support at a certain time. This was David's time and we were here for him.

During my musing, Lawrence came to the kitchen and said, "David wants me to take him to the drug store right away."

I immediately said, "He is too weak. Don't let him go out in this rain."

Lawrence smiled as he squeezed my shoulders and said commandingly, "He wants to go. We will try it."

My shoulders sagged as I realized this might be the beginning of another encounter with a respiratory infection.

Later I found a large, beautiful card on my plate at the luncheon table. Beneath the effusive and emotional printed message was David's own stylized handwritten message: "Although I may not verbalize my appreciation and gratefulness for all you do, know that in my heart I will always love you . . . Dave."

My eyes misted as I hugged and thanked him. He who was created through someone else's love had become mine. I squeezed the thin flesh covering his pointed shoulder blades. His hands came to mine as I nestled my chin in his thinning auburn hair. Frequent, intense discussions between us had bonded us into mutual acceptance. Mere words were unnecessary at this time. There was little we had left unsaid.

I frequently introduced David as "my son." Gradually I became aware that this might be presumptuous, since I knew he had a strong love bond with his biological mother. I did not want to usurp or destroy that. I asked him it if bothered him that I referred to him as "my son."

He quickly replied, "It would bother me a lot more if you didn't."

I was beginning to learn what mothering was all about. I soon realized that the word *mother* is an active verb.

In New York City, David had worked evenings at a hospital a short distance from his apartment. He had his main meal in early afternoon, came home at six o'clock for a snack and break, and had another meal when he came home from work at midnight. He slept most of the forenoon.

Our schedule was quite different. Adult habits do not change easily. We ate our breakfast early. He had his breakfast no earlier than mid morning; that meant he was not hungry when we had lunch at noon but *was* hungry in the afternoon. He frequently ate supper with us, but expected a snack at bedtime and refreshments at midnight.

The schedule in itself was tolerable, but his food needs were the opposite of ours; much of what David ate was forbidden in Lawrence's diet. Most of my time was spent in the kitchen making pastas, egg custards, creamed soups, and puddings. The refrigerator was overcrowded with whole milk and skimmed milk, spicy foods and bland foods, fresh fruit and creamy desserts. The freezer now housed Häagen-Dazs ice cream, ice milk, and sherbet.

David and I spent a lot of time studying cookbooks, looking for recipes for foods he could chew and swallow. His ulcerated mouth not only kept him from talking, but made chewing and swallowing extremely painful. I would ache as I sat across the table from him, watching him struggle to swallow. I waited to see his expression when I served a dish made from a new recipe. Sometimes his eyes lit in appreciation. Occasionally I was drained emotionally because he couldn't eat.

But always, as he walked away from the table, he said, "Thanks, Fran," or, "You tried hard, and I can't eat it. I'm sorry." Invariably we needed to reheat his food (as he would say, "Zap it," in the microwave) because mealtime was a slow, painful process.

I realized how maternal I had become when we were invited to the home of friends who were hosting mutual friends. It seemed important that we accept. The conversation, though stimulating to others, seemed trivial to me. I kept thinking of David and could not enjoy what I considered unimportant and mundane conversation. I realized I was acting like a new mother leaving her firstborn for the first time. I had lost the art of relaxation.

Corporate worship offered reviving spiritual strength. It was there that the words of a nineteenth-century song written by Robert Lowery strengthened me.

My life flows on in endless song,
    above earth's lamentation.
I catch the sweet, though far off hymn
    that hails a new creation.

Through all the tumult and the strife,
    I hear that music ringing,
It finds an echo in my soul.
    How can I keep from singing?

What though my joys and comforts die?
    The Lord my Savior liveth.
What though the darkness gather round?
    Songs in the night he giveth.

The peace of Christ makes fresh my heart,
    a fountain ever springing!
All things are mine, since I am his!
    How can I keep from singing?

And the exhilarating refrain:

No storm can shake my inward calm
    while to that Rock I'm clinging.
Since love is Lord of heav'n and earth,
    how can I keep from singing?

With summer came my birthday—the big, frightening inexpressible seventy which seems to dishearten many. To me it seemed a celebrative milestone. I had made it! Now I had reached the age of utter acceptance. Were not seventy-year-olds allowed to be a bit eccentric? Now, when I forgot something, I could say, "I am seventy years old. What is your excuse?" David and I joked a lot about my new milestone. He needed some smiles! I was ready to be the brunt of his "seventy-ish" humor.

Lawrence had insisted, despite my objections, that we take a break and go to the Buffalo, New York, area for my family reunion. Dan came to stay with Dave. I didn't realize how physically exhausted I was until we left Goshen, and I slept almost the entire 500 miles to my former home community. It was there that I celebrated my birthday. Lawrence had arranged for a surprise cake. It meant much to celebrate this day with my siblings and their families. The tension began to fall away and I was revived. I returned with a new perspective.

During my absence, David had gone to a jewelers and purchased a large, lead-crystal vase. On the card he had written, "To my favorite seventy-year-old, from a grateful son."

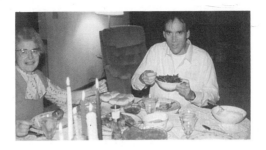

# 7  Living with AIDS

"I saw myself without any clothes on this morning, and I am going to eat you out of house and home!" David grinned as he came to the kitchen, freshly showered and shaved.

I was ready to accept the challenge, as I served the strained oatmeal, fortified with Carnation Instant Breakfast. We tenaciously watched the weight gain for a few weeks, but the discouragement when he lost it so deflated us that we put the scales in the closet. We never mentioned weight again. A part of the dying process devoured all three of us when I needed to make his trousers two inches smaller at the waistline—and when he began buying sweats and lounging clothes because the others were "too stiff and heavy."

It had been a month of adjustments and new experiences, but we were settling in. On his better days David enjoyed going for rides and stopping at unusual stores. He found a large basket which he carefully packed with artifacts and condiments not usually found in the Big Apple. The entire basket was elegantly wrapped and shipped to the office and staff of Doctors Barbara and Sheree Starrett.

We three had been gathering information on AIDS. We had discussed personality and physical changes, knowing that each individual dies at his own pace. We were learning how to say good-bye. While we were buying furnishings for his room, he came to the checkout counter with two visor caps and a pair of fluorescent shoelaces. We both grinned, remembering comments we had read about frivolous purchases. In the deadly serious stage of life, one needs a bit of frivolity to maintain balance. But two caps? And fluorescent shoelaces? He never wore them.

In my journal I wrote,

> That white cap with the wide visor is his constant outdoor companion. He wears it even at the doctor's office. He refuses to use a wheelchair but laboriously plods the long corridors of the hospital to the oncologist's office, keeping that big visor low over his forehead so that he can hardly see where he is going. His head is lowered, apparently embarrassed about the lesions on his face and neck, as if shutting himself from a world of beauty to which he no longer belongs.

David was losing control of his life. He had moved to a new community, away from the friends he had known for twenty years. In Indiana he had no peers and was too weak to develop any close relationships other than family. We needed to think of activities to stimulate him. Joyce Bontrager, the AIDS education nurse, arranged for his attendance at support groups in South Bend. We took rides almost daily.

We planned other activities, but nothing replaced the need for peer relationships. David enjoyed going to Rachel's home, especially in the spring when all the bushes and trees were celebrating new life. But busyness does not replace the innate longing for a close friend. We encouraged him to call his friends, who also called him frequently.

Joyce had planned an AIDS vigil and encouraged us to come. Dave discontinued his IV, and we joined others at the local Presbyterian church. As candles erased the twilight, we prayed for PWAs and their families. We listened to parents who had recently lost a son, heard from an HIV-positive person, and sang "We Shall Overcome." It was a touching hour, and David was deeply moved.

We left quickly. The quietness of the drive home was broken when Dave said, "Dad, will you please drive down to the dam?" We sat there silently while we contemplated the evening. No one spoke until David said, "It's okay. We can go home now." It would be a long night.

At 9:00 a.m. the next morning he was already in the bathroom. My apprehension mounted, for he almost always stayed in his room until after 10. What was wrong now? The dreaded nodes were beginning to appear on his arm which was sore and swollen. He moved slowly. At 10:50 he asked about his 11 a.m. appointment, then realized the appointment was at 4:30 p.m.

David was seen by Dr. Frechen. His hemoglobin

was dangerously low, and he was scheduled to get an infusion of packed red cells the next day.

When he came home, David flopped into his chair. He ate a bit of creamed soup. Discouragement is the final enemy, and he was facing the opponent head-on. David was quiet the rest of the day. Interrupting him seemed to be an invasion. He lay on the davenport, facing the wall, with the IV fluid and medication dripping into his veins. Even with oxygen, he needed to rest during the laborious twenty feet from the davenport to the table.

> May 17, 1991, journal note: That person on the davenport *was* our handsome, ruddy, tall son. Now he is no longer handsome or tall—just long and thin. The absence of fat pads and loss of some hair makes his face look longer. The little finger on his left hand is purple and useless, and he no longer speaks with conviction and force.
>
> He contorts when he swallows, and fills the wastebasket with tissues of drool. His six-foot body is curled in a fetal position, with tubes connected to his chest and nostrils. The virus has depleted him of antibodies, and he has little air passage left for oxygen to get to his lungs.
>
> His entire body is being devoured, and we can only stand by and watch—and cry when he doesn't know it. A part of us gets ripped when we see him suffer.

After his evening meal, I gently rubbed his back and challenged him to a game of Scrabble.

"Dave, I am sorry. All this must be very discouraging."

"Yeah, it's always worse during the night, but in the

morning it doesn't look so bad."

He made a "doze" with the "Z" on the triple word score. I added an "N" to the "doze" and made a vertical "naive" as I asked, "What is it that sustains you?"

There was a long silence. "What is it that sustains me?" he queried.

I waited.

"Well, I guess it's hope."

"Hope in what, David?" I expected that he had gained a new insight into the concept of God. I was eager for his response.

He slowly picked up a tile and said, "Well, hope that somewhere along the long way there will be something that can prolong my life. Hope that they will find a cure for this thing before it is too late."

That response was not what I had wanted to hear. We pushed aside the Scrabble game. Lawrence quickly joined us in one more discussion of faith, trust, hope, and an overwhelming reliance on a God who constantly gives and cares.

Faith and hope were concepts with which David struggled. He had adopted the views of some of the modern theorists who advocate the God within us. Lawrence and I agreed that God is a part of each of us but added our conviction that we are not our own God nor in control of our destiny.

That evening, when my two men retired, I seemed fused to my reclining chair, completely relaxed. The grandfather clock methodically ticked away the precious seconds of life. Such moments of solitude were scarce and sacred. Despite David's illness and prognosis, the past few years had been rich. I was in the right place at the right time. Sometimes one catches a faint insight into the majesty of *being.*

The next day Lawrence stayed with David while he received his packed cells. The infusion had improved his energy and his attitude. When I came back from grocery shopping, Lawrence met me with a "Hi, hon," and David chimed with a "Hi, hon." We had dinner together at a restaurant where the waitress was exceptionally energetic and served our meals efficiently. Dave jokingly commented, "I hope I got some of her blood."

We were on a high but dared not get optimistic. There would be a low. We could only enjoy the moment, knowing more pain would come. Dan called saying he and his family would arrive over the weekend. That thought would sustain Dave until they arrived. Thelma always brought a dietary supplement, which fortified his nutrition.

Beth Landis, a nurse practitioner employed by Dr. Frechen, was God's gift during those hard times. Whenever we had a need, she followed through with appointments. Her competency and caring made her a special family friend. When David was in agony, she arranged for an appointment with a specialist who was leaving in two hours for a vacation in Belgium. Dr. P. called Indianapolis for advice, wrote a prescription and ordered a biopsy.

We were able to get a 5:30 appointment for the biopsy the same day but David waited to see that doctor until 6:30. Waiting was not one of David's gifts. When the doctor did see him, he told David a biopsy would be too dangerous. That meant David had to wait in pain for three more days until his appointment with his oncologist. Yet his will seemed as strong as ever.

An 8:30 appointment in South Bend on Thursday meant that David would need to be up by 6 a.m. We suspected a problem. Lawrence awakened him. He left without breakfast but was still fifteen minutes late for his appointment. Dr. S. was concerned that he hadn't seen Dr. T. recently and made arrangements for Dave to see him in Goshen at 5:00 that afternoon. Dr. T. recommended that Dave see Dr. P. in South Bend for a biopsy at 5:00 p.m. the next day. (David was seen by five different doctors that week.)

By this time, David should have known how long it took to drive to South Bend, especially in Friday afternoon traffic. A half hour before we planned to leave for the appointment with Dr. P., our tension mounted when we heard him in the shower.

We waited. His dad knocked on the bathroom door. "Dave, we need to leave in a few minutes." No response. We waited. We wondered what we could do to make him move faster. After we waited more tense moments, he came. I held the door open, trying not to show my disgust. Lawrence was waiting in the car with the motor running. It was a troubled, quiet thirty-mile ride.

At the hospital the elevator seemed unusually slow. When we got to Dr. P.'s office twenty minutes late, there was a note on the door for David Greaser, telling him to go to the emergency room. Medical people, like everyone else, like to get off on schedule, especially on Fridays. David's tension now matched mine. We raced through the halls, asking any person-

nel we could find how to get to the emergency room—
four stories and many corridors below us.

When we arrived at last, another doctor, who did
not know David, incised the lesion for the biopsy. David had to fill out new papers and pay the emergency
room bill. There was continued silence on the way
home, but we hoped he had learned a bit about
promptness. Two days later, when we left for a social
appointment, he asked, "Am I being rushed again?"

David, who had lived independently, could not
easily adjust to the schedule of others. He seemed to
think that medical people were usually behind schedule and saw no reason to be prompt for appointments.
We, on the other hand, forgot too quickly that a poor
blood count does not allow one to move with the am-
bition many of us have. His hemoglobin continued to
be sub-normal, despite blood transfusions, and his T4
cell count, which should have been between 800 and
1,000 was 60. We needed to apologize for our own in-
sensitivities.

The tensions of the seesaw of emotions, coupled
with the many appointments and the anxiety of wondering what else we could do, had its effect on Lawrence. He began complaining about pain in his chest.
Knowing that stress is a major cause of heart attacks, I
became weak and angry at Dave. Was I, in my concern
for his nutrition, neglecting Lawrence's dietary needs?

Anxieties began to cripple my effectiveness. We
immediately arranged for testing. I expected to be
chastised for not watching his diet more closely. In my
emotional turmoil, I leaned over the kitchen sink and
cried, "Oh, God, if you have to take one, don't let it be

Lawrence." Tests assured us the chest pain was stress-related.

David's spirits were rising. His brother Galen from Texas, and his friend Glenn Andersson from New York City were coming for a few days. David needed to acquaint Glenn with his new community. Galen, who had entertained them in Texas, was a good host to introduce Glenn to Indiana.

On Sunday Glenn went to church with us and seemed to enjoy the worship service. Rachel and her family and Grandma came for Sunday dinner. Everyone participated in the laughter and free-flowing conversation. David was obviously enjoying the day. I watched Glenn's face as he interacted. An only child without a father and with a confused mother, he was obviously yearning for the joy a family could bring. This only made him feel more sorry for Dave. In a pensive mood, he later commented to me, "Dave has so much going for him—all this plus a family. Why couldn't it have been me instead of Dave who got AIDS?" To this day Glenn is HIV-negative.

Glenn and I were early risers, so we sat at the patio table drinking coffee while he told me his story. We talked seriously about his experience with homosexuality, the rejection he felt from his cousins, David's AIDS, and his own ideas of spirituality. He had enjoyed our worship service and knew our minister came weekly to see David. Glenn needed a counselor, a listener, and a family. He began to feel as if he belonged to this community and looked forward to bringing his mother here.

It appeared that the roller coaster was again

headed down. David complained of a sore throat and mouth. Pureed, creamed non-acidic soups seemed to be the only foods he could tolerate, except for ice cream and egg custard. Though he blamed his exhaustion on a new medication, I blamed it on overexertion. Lawrence and I had agreed that we would not restrict his activity, even if he **would** listen to us. He deserved to be happy, whether or not it meant an earlier death.

David saw Dr. Frechen. Since the two were alone, we didn't know what was said, but he came home discouraged. Talking was not easy at any time. He missed his social group but we could not create friendships for him. Fighting death is a losing battle, but we kept trying. He was back to written messages again.

It was 10:30 a.m. and David was still in his room, undoubtedly with a concern similar to mine. What other solution could we try to ease the pain of swallowing? The nutritionist from CareMark called, but she had no suggestions we had not already tried.

Dave came out looking like a lonely orphan. "I'm weak, short of breath, and depressed."

"Dave, do you need a hug?"

"I sure do!"

Later he came to the kitchen and thanked me for the hug.

Our pleasant days were over. David had a burning sore throat, ate almost no lunch, and declared that he was not going to take any medication or eat anything until his throat cleared. The situation became more tense when the doctor did not return our call. He finally took oral medication, waited, then ate sparingly.

On a misty afternoon, when the sun and rain vied

for supremacy, the rain was winning. Despite David's pain, he needed to find a specific compact disc case to house the extensive library of CDs he had already given to his father. We tried many stores, but the style he wanted was not available.

I tried to convince him that the gift he had already bought was enough for Father's Day. He replied indignantly, "Fran, *it is not!*" Despite his different lifestyle, he had a deep respect for his father. We never did find what he wanted, but he settled for an appropriate card. There was no conversation on the way home.

> June 17 journal entry: Oh, God, are we starting another difficult siege? He coughed a lot last night, and now he appears to have a fever. Some of this is expected if he isn't eating enough, but do we have to go through this again? How long will this last? How much stamina do we need? Where is help?
>
> We must be courageous for him. He is already living on determination and an amazingly strong self-strength. We would be ready to let him go if we could be sure of his belief in you. Yet maybe he knows you in ways I don't understand. He has deep respect for a supreme being and all the created beings.
>
> Do I need to accept his faith as sufficient? Is mine sufficient? He seems to have knowledge of your love. But is he ready to believe that it is for him?

I served him ground chicken, strained corn, and applesauce along with fresh tapioca pudding. He tried valiantly to eat, but in half an hour he was chilled and vomited everything. We were all discouraged. In my dejection, I thought of Edna St. Vincent Millay's poem, "When It Is Over."

> When it is over—for it will be over,
> Though we who watch it be gone,
> watched it and with it died. . . .

I silently rubbed his back, then hugged him. His body relaxed in my embrace as he said, "I wanted a hug yesterday, but you were too busy." *God, forgive me if I ever pretend I am too busy to be available!*

Beth arranged for lab work and more packed cells. While David was receiving blood, Lawrence and I had a lovely dinner along a relaxing lake, thirty miles away, far enough to ventilate the mind and get a different perspective. How difficult it would be to be alone in this assignment! A drive around the lake reminded us of the beauty which surrounded us, if we took time to see it.

I remembered that God seldom created new resources for people. He simply opened their eyes. He didn't create the well just for the dying widow; he opened her eyes. So often our strength and need is supplied from sources already close to us. We only need our eyes opened to see it. We saw beauty around us and were refreshed for whatever would lie ahead. When we picked up David at the hospital and told him where we had been, he jokingly chided us for taking advantage of his absence. He knew we needed it.

Our pleasant days were beginning again. A trip to the blueberry marsh was a spiritual experience for David. On the way home, we stopped in silence as we watched an Amish barn raising. That kind of community support was difficult for a city-bred person to understand, and he was impressed.

The oxygen machine had changed its status. I previously saw it as an impostor and was weakened when Dave needed it. Later, its gentle bubbling became a lullaby of life support for which I was grateful.

Nights were especially long for David. It became routine to awaken at 3:00 a.m. and check to see if David's light was on. He was often in the living room watching television, trying to get his mind off reality. Lawrence ordered cable television so he could have a greater variety of programs.

I cried inwardly as I planted the pansies he bought for me. I know he wanted to dig in the earth, but instead he sat inside the patio door and watched as I asked him where I should plant them.

I noticed that he did not take his IV pole in his bedroom that evening and wondered what that meant. He would obviously not be taking his IV antibiotic. Was he giving up?

June 21 journal entry: I am beginning to resonate with the tens of thousands of mothers who have watched that pernicious virus eat away at the live flesh which was once part of their body. One can do all the physical gestures of nourishing and the emotional gestures of nurturing, but can only stand by and watch as the body gradually becomes debilitated and is eventually conquered by the vicious killer . . . and the killer always wins.

Dear God, oh, dear God, sudden death would be so much easier.

David awoke with a burning sore throat and ate no lunch. He wrote his messages to me. We both grinned when I started to write my answers. He was seen by the oncologist, who expressed dismay at the lesion in his throat, which he declared (with an expletive) was a "big hole the size of a quarter." David was going to South Bend daily for cobalt therapy to his arm, yet his arm seemed to be no better.

Later he pulled his body into fetal position on the davenport; his skinny arms, big at the elbows, stuck out like gnarled knots on a tree. There were no words.

"Dave," I timidly asked, "are you giving up?"

He shook his head.

There seemed to be no medication to control the mouth ulcers. It was a difficult day. In the evening he took his medication and came to the kitchen for food but was uncomfortably quiet. Then someone called to invite me for lunch. It seemed uncanny that during the deepest discouragement, someone would offer some special nicety.

After an exhausting trip to a nature park in Michigan, David poured out his loneliness. Going to a support group was discouraging. The few who were there were still in the denial stage. (*Did I hear right, Dave? Isn't that what you used to say?*) Another time when he tried the support group again, the driver did not show, so he wasn't attending anymore. We could not replace peers, but we could be friends.

Rachel and her family suggested that Dave go with them for a weekend with their brother Dan in Ohio. Dave hesitated but decided to go. Although he came home exhausted, the experience gave him peer and sibling stimulation.

The break was good for Lawrence and me. Our

emotions had been strained to breaking. When one is emotionally exhausted, one becomes oversensitive, and every word can be misconstrued. Lawrence was as tense as I, and we could both be hurt by comments which under other circumstances would be easily accepted.

I wallowed in self-pity. Sometimes I got angry at David. We missed our Sunday school retreat but wanted to be home with David. We purposely did not put it on the calendar so he would not see it and insist that we go. A visitor asked if we were going. David was hurt that we were "sacrificing." I would have enjoyed entertaining guests in our home, but David's unpredictable health ruled that out. Lawrence was unable to go golfing with his friends because of David's appointments. Lawrence would not consider golfing if David needed him.

I privately wished for my study/sewing room but David needed it. I enjoyed stretching out on the davenport occasionally, but David had made that his daybed. I missed my corner of the study for my "centering" time every morning.

But I was consciously aware that God was with me and hearing me wherever I worshiped. Despite moodiness, I felt the strong support of myriads of prayers. My life flowed on "in endless song above earth's lamentations."

My self-pity eventually dissipated. David wanted to live, ride a bicycle against the wind, plant more trees, pick roses, and absorb the sun along the lake. We wanted all these for him, so our petty sacrifices were minimal. Taking care of him was our privilege.

It had always been planned that if David ever came home, he would use the lower level of our house, where he could be undisturbed and have more privacy. His condition made that impossible, but he did enjoy an occasional slow trek to the basement. As he plodded his way up the steps, he told me there was a spider in the bathroom.

"Oh, I hope you killed it."

He grinned. "No."

I should have known he wouldn't, for David would not be unkind to any person or creature.

On return trips from chemotherapy, father and son often took back roads and scanned cemeteries. David had definite ideas about his burial site. They checked the old part of a local cemetery with the sexton, who showed them available lots. As he was talking, David wandered to a spot along the river near a tree. The sexton said that it was not a marked gravesite but there would be room for one body. Dave quickly responded, "I want it!"

I heard the garage doors open as they drove in. Dave climbed the one step into the kitchen, leaned against the wall, grinned triumphantly, and said, "Fran, I lucked out!" Excitedly he told me about his gravesite.

David now seemed to be on a plateau. He came to the kitchen one morning grinning.

"It's good to see you smiling, Dave. Is something funny?"

The smile lit his eyes "Nothing hurts!"

"You mean your mouth isn't sore?"

"Oh, sure, it's still sore, but nothing else hurts. It's amazing!"

I continued doing the laundry.

He followed me to the doorway. "I'm wondering, Fran. What are the odds of you making me some cornbread?"

It was going to be a good day.

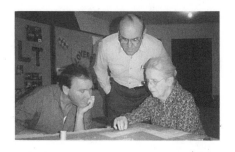

# 8 AIDS and the Faith Community

AIDS has wrapped its gruesome tentacles around the entire world. It has killed millions, destroyed families, and created orphans. It continues to maim and frighten society. Unfortunately, AIDS will be with us for a long time. It is one of the more serious health problems the world has faced. According to the World Health Organization, by the year 2000, 39 million adults and 10 million children worldwide will be infected by the HIV virus believed to cause AIDS. Forty million is equivalent to the population of Canada and Australia combined.

The United States Department of Health and Human Services estimated that in 1993 one million Americans were infected with HIV. Three million persons were infected worldwide. One hundred thousand persons have died of AIDS in the United States. The first one hundred thousand cases worldwide were reported over an eight-year period; the second one hundred thousand in just twenty-six months.

In January 1994, the definition of AIDS was expanded to include pulmonary tuberculosis, recurrent pneumonia, and some types of cancer. In addition, according to the Center for Disease Control (CDC) a lessening of the body's master immune cells (called CD4s) to 200 per cubic millimeter, or one-fifth of normal, would mean the person has acquired immune deficiency syndrome.

AIDS seems most prevalent among adults aged twenty-five to forty-four. In the United States, the HIV infection rate is increasing four times faster in women than in men. An increasing number of children are left orphaned by this killer. During 1991, according to the Mayo Clinic Health Letter and CDC publications, AIDS among teenagers increased 77 percent. In 1993, CDC reported that more than thirty four thousand people over fifty had full-blown AIDS—more than double the figure reported the previous year.

The virus causing AIDS enters the blood and quickly penetrates certain white cells, called T4 cells. The white cells are the body's infection-fighting cells. The virus attaches itself to the cell and passes on its own genetic material. HIV cells are produced and live in the host cell. As this happens, the person's resistance to infection becomes weaker, for the white cells are being destroyed. As it passes through the blood stream, HIV infects other T4 cells, which lose their infection-fighting power.

Unable to fight infections due to a weakened immune system, a person with AIDS becomes more susceptible to opportunistic infections. The virus can affect any organ of the body—heart, lungs, eyes, kidney, or brain. Regardless of what parts of the body are affected, the person with AIDS faces major physical and emotional changes. The symptoms vary, but all AIDS sufferers experience isolation, loneliness, and, in too many cases, the killing pain of rejection.

Despite the ugly Kaposi (cancer) sores, the sore mouth and throat which causes drooling, the difficult breathing, or the physical and emotional changes, the personhood of the sufferer is still intact. The basic human needs are the same. He or she is still a child of God, who needs to experience God's love and care from us.

AIDS is not a "we-they" illness. It is an "us" illness. Until a cure for AIDS is found, all of us will live with this robber. But there is a social illness for which we have a cure. The symptoms are judgmentalism, fear, disgrace, shame, rejection, and isolation. The cure for the symptoms is freely available through Christ, who offers compassion, love, care, and forgiveness. While we wait for a medical cure, we can busy ourselves eliminating intolerance and needless suffering. The love of Christ overwhelmingly accepts all people, regardless of the origin of their pain. It is our responsibility to love and to show that love through nonjudgmental caring.

Persons with AIDS present a challenge and opportunity to exemplify Christ's caring. Christ chose to alleviate pain, rather than making discretionary judgments about who deserved his care. When Christ healed the man of his blindness, he did not do a study on *why* he was blind, even though society would expect that in that day. Nor did Christ heal only those who agreed with his new message. His retort, to the disciples' surprise, was that the sick are the ones who need a doctor, not the well ones. In the same vein, we need to stop asking how a PWA became infected. Christ's example points to healing, not to etiology.

I was reminded of this when I had nagging questions as to whether David *really* got the virus from a needle prick, as he so adamantly insisted. I doubted any person so exhausted would have had the strength to insist on an untruth. I needed to believe him, but I expressed my doubts to a special doctor friend.

The friend immediately responded, "Fran, it doesn't matter *how* he got it. Right now he needs your love and care."

After that, the origin of David's AIDS was not an issue. We never discussed it further.

The AIDS crisis is an opportunity for the church to model the caring of Christ. Instead of asking how someone got infected, we need to ask what God wants us to do to help. AIDS has a ripple effect and touches many lives. All people involved with AIDS make their greatest contribution when they meet on a common ground—one person greatly loved by God meeting another person equally loved and valued by God.

Many PWAs are reaching out in their search for meaning and ultimately find God. Some find it difficult to consider a God in the midst of suffering, because some people who claim to love God have rejected PWAs. Many have felt ostracized and rejected in the name of God and the church.

Some become cynical as they watch friends die, and ask, "If there is a God of love, why is this allowed?" That cynicism has sometimes been strengthened by New Age streams of thought which stress the God within each of us and self-empowerment. Many others have turned to God and have found internal healing and fortitude.

However, it is hard to accept God's universal love when one feels the condemnation of God's people. If God's people are not available to give hope and show a way of love, those suffering will continue to look to other sources, including self-empowerment, meditation, spiritism, massage, and communication with the dead.

Ministering in Christ's name is the free gift of self to others, reflecting God's free gift to us. If caring is done solely in an attempt to evangelize, it is not a ministry and can be counterproductive. Caring is our opportunity to represent God's unconditional love for all humans. It is God's business to "save" PWAs.

The church must continue to grapple with the theological and ethical issues in the context of the AIDS crisis. The questions are sometimes ambiguous and the answers unsatisfactory, but we must continue to struggle. To do nothing makes a strong statement and can be deadly. The crisis is everyone's crisis and cannot be postponed. We must share in the solution.

The challenge of AIDS is for the church to be God's agent of love and reconciliation to the world. David Hallman, editor of *AIDS Issues: Confronting the Challenge* (Pilgrim Press, 1989), says:

> The church must share in this experience, changing and being changed so as to enable society to provide a sup-

portive presence for those who are grieving and suffering. The church must become part of the AIDS pilgrimage to deeper understanding: it must join the journey toward human wholeness.

The word *heal* is related to the word *whole*, which itself is derived from the German word *heilig*, meaning "holy" or "hallowed." The healing process is one of becoming whole again.

AIDS, surprisingly, can become a gift. Many, once they have learned of their death sentence, have set goals for their lives and made unique contributions. Some have recognized, almost too late, that life is a gift, and have begun to live it in celebration. Some have learned new appreciation for the value of friendship, one of the greatest blessings.

One PWA, now deceased, said, "We feel connected with all living things. Vision becomes more acute. We see new shades of blue and green, and, ah, yellow daffodils!" Another reported, "We begin to notice and live in the moment. And when we notice, we somehow know that the world was made for love." Another PWA noted, "I am a better person since I have the disease. I am more focused." One said, "For twenty years I didn't have a life. Now I'm in a hurry to put a whole lifetime into the time I have left."

Can AIDS actually be a gift? These are some of the gifts we learned: In the midst of grief's strangling grip, the prayers of caring friends renewed our spirits and sustained us with an inner calm and strength.

We learned that to face death realistically is to begin to live. We learned that it is important to give *now*.

We learned to place greater value on relationships and to nurture them reverently.

We learned that faith is not blind acceptance. Faith is a truth nurtured through exposure, which eventually jells into a conviction.

We learned that a blind faith is not faith at all. Faith, to be real, must be tested and personally avowed.

We learned that the richness of a Christian community is God's precious gift, to be nurtured and enjoyed.

We learned through our many supportive friends that those who have suffered are the most compassionately caring.

We learned that *today* is a special moment, a gift which is free. Today is ours to see, smell, hear, and touch. Today is ours to show God's love in caring ways.

We learned that beauty can be found in unexpected places. We need to look deeper or develop keener eyesight, but beauty surrounds us.

We learned that life, during the night, can be very discouraging, but in the morning, everything looks better.

Tragedy can be a wedge which separates or draws people closer. It is our choice. AIDS can exacerbate an existing problem or help resolve it. AIDS helped us have three beautiful years with David we might otherwise not have experienced. AIDS helped us establish priorities and be realistic about important life-and-death issues.

AIDS taught us to focus on *living* while knowing that death is part of the continuum.

AIDS allowed us to take risks. It meant knowing what we wanted from life, and what we wanted to give.

When we were deprived of what we had before, we began to realize how much we had to enjoy. Together we learned that life can be more beautiful than before.

David learned what we already knew: that God's love and forgiveness, which is revealed through God's children, brings peace, acceptance, healing, and deep gratitude.

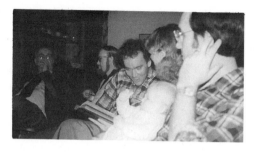

# 9 Doubts and Faith

"When it is over, and after I am buried," he said, looking at me with a grin he hoped I would understand, "I'd like everyone to go back to the church. I want to treat them to a meal. We'll have it catered. I'd like to do that."

"David, the church will take care of that. We always do that for the family when someone dies." His special gift was squelched, but the overwhelming concept of the church continuing its gift of love even after death was still amazing him. "It's important in the grieving process that we all be together. You'll be with us in spirit. We need to do this before we go our separate ways again."

Dying was not an unusual subject. We knew death would happen sometime. He knew now that, despite his bravado, finally he would lose. We could not shake that grim reality.

The lawyer and his secretary came to legalize and witness David's legal power of attorney. Most arrange-

ments had been made. His casket was chosen and purchased. He was prepared for his death. It was the dying that was elusive and frightening.

Yet the gift of hope gave him comfort and courage.
Without hope, one is already dead. But without suffering, there would be no need for hope. Now even hope
was becoming harder to grasp. When in all the travail
of daily deterioration does one allow hope to ebb?

I remembered, with a tinge of a pained conscience,
our conversation as we studied nutritious, easily swal-
lowed foods. David rinsed his mouth after every attempt to speak. "Why don't you take some more mor-
phine, Dave?

"I took some an hour ago." He slowly put down his
glass.

"Take more, Dave. You might as well be comfortable." I lowered my voice, "You aren't going to be able
to cure this anyway."

He stopped abruptly, looked directly at me and an-
grily said, "What is *that* supposed to mean?" He almost
snarled as he said it.

I looked at him just as squarely. "We all know it's
terminal. We can't stop it anymore. Stay comfortable."

Was it cruel of me to say that, or was I helping him
face the ultimate reality? Comfort was more important
than combat when there was no cure, I reasoned with
myself. Or should I have continued to give him hope,
despite all the signs of defeat?

David was quiet for the rest of the evening. Talking
of serious issues required energy he no longer had.
Yet we needed to talk. Would he find faith before he
gave up? Should we maintain hope, despite the pain of

a situation where hope no longer was indicated?

Weeks earlier, when we came home from church, David had asked, "Couldn't we invite Axel here for a meal with us?" It was not unusual for David to be sensitive to another's need. What secretly delighted us was that David had listened to our church's worship service by radio and heard the announcement that Axel, a Central American refugee, was being welcomed into our church community.

We began noticing that our church periodicals were rearranged. Apparently he was reading them during the night or while we were away. We deliberately left some pertinent literature within easy reach on the coffee table. He read with interest the reader's responses to issues on homosexuality in our denominational paper. That the church was even discussing the issue, controversial though it might be, he saw as a surge of freedom.

David felt liberated by open discussion of the secret he had felt he had to keep hidden all his life. It was powerful for him to be accepted for something he believed he could not control. Yet like so many of God's provisions, the resources and love he needed had been available all the time. David's expectations of being rejected had limited his ability to feel accepted and had narrowed his concept of God.

David recognized the different viewpoints on the homosexual issue and respected those who disagreed with him. But he was angry at pious preachers who insisted that AIDS was God's curse on homosexuals.

Never had we been so aware of the amount of energy it takes to read. Friends suggested and brought appropriate books, but thinking was exhausting. We became acquainted with new authors.

I shared with David the insights I learned from books by Frederick Buechner, who shares profound concepts in a lucid style. Too late I encountered, in *Awakened from Within*, the insights of Brother Roger of Taize', who notes that accepting our doubts creates a greater readiness to accept the truth. I needed to be reminded that understanding is more important than being understood. Brother Roger also consoled me by reminding me that even Dostoyevsky in his Siberian prison admitted to disbelief, and doubt because of his thirst to believe.

Had I been stifling both David's and my spiritual growth by my attempts to fit him into my myopic version of God? My own doubts surfaced, but I did not reveal them. Had I deprived him of opportunities for growth through my deception?

I could not doubt God's love, for love was incarnated in people who surrounded us. As long as David was with us, he must be allowed to mature in his own version of faith—just as we would in ours. Faith is not faith until it is tested, and its condition must be personally examined. This can only be done if we are honest and understand that no one else can examine our faith for us. I could not determine the condition of David's faith. I could only trust God for that. "For who among men knows the thoughts of man except the man's spirit within him" (1 Cor. 2:11).

We would continue to put our trust in God and allow God to bring David to faith. This was our opportunity to love. God would receive the fruit of that love.

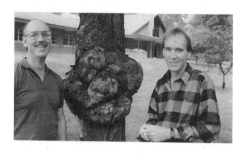

# **10** And a Time to Die

It was going to be an exciting week for David. Both Galen and Glenn would be arriving for another visit, and David was hoping to accompany them to the well-publicized September Michiana Mennonite Relief Sale. Over 30,000 people from many states would be converging at the fairgrounds for a Mennonite Central Committee sale. All proceeds—over half a million dollars—would go for worldwide relief from suffering.

To be energized for the occasion, David was again getting packed cells. Glenn arrived earlier than expected but enjoyed helping us eat leftovers. He needed the treasure of being a family member around the kitchen table.

Galen, who arrived the next day, has the ability to make any occasion a jubilant time. It was good to see the trio enjoying all the activities the community provided. David dared not miss any opportunity to acquaint them with his new environment. They came back from a preview of the sale with glowing reports and many purchases. Tomorrow would be a full day.

A pancake-and-sausage breakfast at the sale was too great a temptation to miss. It was agreed that Lawrence would go with them, and I would bring David later. Knowing that David would sleep late, I began baking bread. By 10:00 a.m. he was dressed and mildly insisting that we leave immediately. The yeast was left to do its leavening, for I was sure we would not stay long.

We began the long slow walk to the quilt building, where David found his family. With a bidding number in his hand, he watched the sale of every quilt. Would a quilt purchase be another evidence of "frivolous" spending? By 3:00 p.m. I was ready to leave and take him with me. He wanted to stay. The bread was a total loss.

David showed no evidence of exhaustion as ten of us laughed and told stories around the supper table. Any physical strain he endured that day was worth the pain it might cause later. The lively discussion in the living room entertained me as I baked pies at 11:00 p.m. How good for Dave to be able to relate to peers! Next week may be difficult, but at least he had had the weekend.

Rachel and her family and Grandma joined us for a "fatted calf" dinner the next day. I voiced no objection to Glenn's insistence that he make dinner on Monday evening. Lawrence and he shopped for gourmet foods, while David set the table with our best linen, china, and crystal. Candlelight added a celebrative aura to the happy occasion. David was having no pain and was surrounded by those he loved most.

Then it was time for Galen to return to Texas. Lawrence suggested that we take him to Chicago for his flight, and we stay overnight. "That would give us a break while Glenn is here with Dave." The fellows gave their strong approval, and I offered no resistance. Those two days of unhurried and unworried relaxation were a wondrous gift of rejuvenation.

When we returned, Glenn was preparing the evening meal and would not allow me in the kitchen. All of us became engrossed in a discussion of activities during our absence. David and Glenn had driven to Shipshewana where, among other things, David bought an antique wind-up train which he "had always wanted under the Christmas tree."

The three men became little boys again as they sprawled on the rug, releasing adult inhibitions and enjoying the wonder of the miniature train. We also learned that Glenn had had car trouble and that, amazingly, David had driven our car on a busy highway so he could pick up Glenn at the garage.

David was on a high, for Glenn had decided to stay until the weekend. We wanted David to enjoy the moments, although we did not look forward to the descent. His energy level did ebb, and by Friday he was ready to stay at home, where he and Glenn made impressive dried flower arrangements from the huge supply they brought back from a country ride. Reminiscing about activities and friends in New York City was a frequent activity.

Early Saturday morning we noticed a light in the living room. David was on the davenport gasping for breath. Our attempts to relax him failed. The oxygen machine was no longer an adequate provider. Apprehension shone out of his narrowed eyes, and his skin was clammy. His rapid but thready pulse told us he was in crisis; oxygen was not getting to his lungs. He needed more help than we could give him at home.

Glenn heard the commotion and joined in our concern. David vacillated between wanting to go to the hospital and wanting to stay home. It was the weekend, and both his doctor and Beth, his nurse practitioner, were on vacation.

Then frantically David said, "Fran, if I don't get to the hospital soon, it's curtains for me!"

We took him to the emergency room. He was admitted to the care of a doctor who had never seen him.

Was this the end? It was true—regardless of our readiness to die, when the actual time seems to have arrived, we desperately hang on.

Tubes and machines were attached to his arms and chest. On his chart were listed over twenty medications. Therapies were begun.

Was this really what David wanted? Discouragement rose. Did we dare hope for more time together? How many financial and medical resources should be invested in this terminal illness? How much was a day of life worth?

Glenn was also in turmoil, vacillating between reality and desire, for it was time for him to return to his hallucinating mother, but he wanted to be with David.

By Tuesday, Glenn knew he had to leave. It was no longer safe to leave his mother alone. David's test results were coming back. He had three kinds of pneumonia and would be placed in reverse isolation to protect him from incoming bacteria.

Dr. T. came to David and discussed the gravity of the situation and David's living will. Did David want to reconsider and have intubation? David needed to think about that overnight. He wrestled with the decision during the restless midnight hours. In the morning he told Dr. T. he would abide by his living will. He wanted no resuscitation. Regardless of how well one prepares for death, the work of dying is sometimes painful.

Six months after bringing David to our home, we sat by his hospital bedside counting the pulsations, even as we cherished the minutes. Lawrence was suffering the pain of a father losing a son.

For the first time since admission three days before, David was relaxed. In his attempt to sleep, his yellowed lip hung limply as he gasped to breathe.

"David, can you hear me?" I asked. "I need to tell you that your life has mattered very much. The world around you has become better because you touched it. I still don't understand it all, but I have dropped any judgments against you. I love you as a child of God. Your appreciation of a voice of God you found in people and nature transcended my small world. My knowledge of God has grown because of you."

Mostly we sat by silently, hoping. Hoping for what? Release? Improvement? Possibly a bit more time of clarity when we could discuss our relationships with an overwhelmingly loving God.

Earlier that day, Rachel had talked to David about God and said, "If you believe, squeeze my hand." There was a slight twitch. Was that all he could do? Or all he wanted to do? The answer is with God. We entrusted him to God's love. We could do no more.

David's oral sores had cleared, but his weakness limited our conversation. His T cells were virtually nonexistent. Strength-giving platelets were being absorbed but rapidly devoured by the AIDS monster.

It was obvious that David had exhausted himself at the Relief Sale and all the other activities which he and Glenn enjoyed afterward. It was a dear price, but we had no regrets. If he died, he would have enjoyed himself to death.

I remembered the time he was laboriously panting as he ascended the basement steps. I grinned. "Statistically, every time you climb stairs you add two seconds to your life, so keep climbing!"

He replied, "But if it takes me ten minutes to save two seconds, it's still a losing battle."

I wondered if those two seconds would help him now. His doctor was efficient and knowledgeable and seemed to be doing everything possible to save him. But despite the medications, cultures, and therapies, his lungs did not clear.

We who had been praying, "Don't die!' were now saying, "God, take him." There was healing in the midst of dying. He was a child again, and in those voiceless days, he would reach for a hand and be grateful for our presence.

An ominous phone call startled us at 2:45 on Thursday morning. The nurse from the hospital said, "David is having a restless night. He thinks he's dying. He wants you here."

It is a haunting sensation to go to a hospital in the

eerie predawn hours, when the whole community is wrapped in penetrating stillness. The elevator seemed excessively slow. The halls were silent and there was little activity. We wore gowns and masks as we reached for David's hands.

David's eyes were big and frightened as he reached for us. He exclaimed, "I'm terrified! I think I'm dying!" We pulled the curtain and touched where we could, around all the tubes attached to him.

"It's okay, Dave." Our heads almost touched his as we softly talked. "Just relax and let it happen. It's okay to die."

He lifted his head and stared at us incredulously and asked, "It's okay to die?" as if saying, "This is no time to tease. This is serious!"

"Yes, David, it's okay. Just relax and let it happen. It's all right."

His head relaxed on the pillow. We stood by, holding and touching. His eyelids closed while we quoted the Shepherd Psalm. His father started the tape recorder; strains of the *Messiah* filled the room. We prayed. We hummed hymns. We told him how much God and we loved him.

We watched the color of his fingernails fade from pink to pale and then blue. We watched the area around his mouth become white. We held his hands and felt his pain when his mouth contorted to gasp, for his lungs were too full of fluid to allow him the luxury of breathing. We felt the thready pulse until there was no pulse to feel.

We said our good-byes to him. Finally we stopped. Life was gone. At that moment we were on sacred ground. We knew we had witnessed something holy.

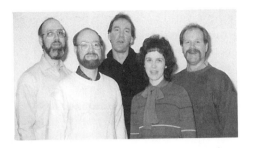

# 11 Afterword

Despite our diminished family, there was no diminishing of community support. Barbara came as soon as she heard. After her hug of condolence, she immediately began dusting the basement before she left for her employment. Telephone messages of sympathy and promises of food were blessing us. The children and the extended family began arriving.

Numerous phone calls from David's friends in New York City reminded us of the impact David's life had on theirs. Glenn was grief-stricken, for he found it impossible to leave his confused mother alone. Lawrence's sister stayed close to her mother during Grandma's grieving. Though exhausted, I was tearless. We had done our grieving as we did what we could for David's well-being. David was now totally in God's hands.

Amid the pain of David's leaving, there came an undeniable sigh of relief. His suffering was done. No longer need he struggle to be strong enough to face the probability of dying a few months or weeks later. Now it was time to celebrate his life through remembering.

Family and close friends were with us at the prayer service at the funeral home. Steve Chupp, pastor of Zion Chapel, where Rachel and her family worship, told us of his hospital conversation with David. Steve had told Dave about a video he had recently seen which talked of God's wonderful act of creating all things in nature as well as all humanity. Then he asked Dave, "Are you ready to meet this God?"

David asked, "But how can I know he is *really* there?" David was ready, interested, and eager for a discussion.

David had pushed the God of his youth out of his life. Now he was trying to convince himself his reasons for rejecting that God remained valid. "But," Steve continued, "the God he ignored seemed so real to him in the lives of those who cared for him. He wanted that same reality. If it was real for them, he wanted that reality for himself."

For the past twenty years, David had argued against God. More recently, he struggled with facing God in his present condition. He was non-argumentative, simply struggling, Steve reported.

Pastor Steve's words were not the ones usually heard at a prayer service, but they comforted us. Pastor Waltner had a brief meditation and prayer, and the family gathered around Dave in a final farewell. Each of us put a flower on his lifeless body before the coffin lid shut him forever from our view.

The mourning caravan made a solemn trip to the

burial site along the river. We again held flowers from David's many love-gifts as we heard "to dust thou shalt return." David would have liked that. This was his opportunity to become one with the nature he had so enjoyed.

The service was over, but no one wanted to leave. Words were unnecessary as we silently prayed and enjoyed the beauty of the setting and listened to the rippling river. Galen spontaneously suggested that we sing "I'm gonna lay down my burdens down by the riverside."

We tried. But sadness and song do not blend well. Amid his tears, Galen suggested we try it again. This time we sang more triumphantly: "I'm gonna lay down my burdens down by the riverside. Ain't gonna suffer here no more!"

That bittersweet experience turned a mournful moment into a celebrative event. David was finished with suffering and had moved to a new experience.

◊ ◊ ◊

It was time for our diminished family to strengthen bonds through tears, laughter, reminiscing, and appreciating. Relatives from other states helped make it a wholesome family event. David would have been so grateful to know that his cousin Steve had come from New York to mourn and celebrate with us.

We scheduled the public memorial service as a Sunday vesper service. At dusk, when the ethereal meets the earthly, we were again buoyed by the many friends who joined us in the celebration of David's life.

One large, ivy-entwined candle gave witness to the light he had shed, while flowers stood as sentinels to his memory.

David's Aunt Frances set a worshipful tone when she played organ renditions of hope and beauty. Pastor Waltner read the "blesseds" from Matthew 5. So many seemed befitting to David: "Blessed are the merciful . . . the meek . . . poor in spirit . . . hungering and thirsting after righteousness."

Family members had prepared their letters to David. Dan tried to constrain his emotions as he said,

"It is at times like this that we think about family and those who have gone before us. I think of Grandma and Grandpa Troyer, of Grandpa Greaser, and of my mother. Then I think of their many qualities and the generosity with which they shared, their unselfishness, their caring for others, and caring for their families. Their endurance and their patience stand out in my mind. They acted on their convictions.

"Then I think of my brother Dave. It is this heritage which is most important and is an exemplary message for us. I know that if David were here, he would want to give special thanks to Dad and Fran for their nurture, love, and care—and for their acceptance of what and who he was.

"I want to give special thanks to Steve Troyer, who was like a brother to David when the rest of us were unable to be there.

"If David were here, he would want us to continue to reach out to people in the way he did, especially to those who now and in the future find themselves victims of AIDS. I hope that we who have gone through this experience are better equipped with compassion, courage, and love for those who are hurting. If we act in this form of service, we will be fulfilling in part the heritage and the example passed on by our foreparents and by my brother David."

Uncle Dana and Aunt Verna read the other prepared statements. None of us were capable of speaking coherently in public. Tears surfaced too easily.

◖◗ ◖◗ ◖◗

*Rachel's letter to Dave*
Dave, you will always be a special big brother to me. You were the one who heard a neighbor calling me, using a Spanish accent. From then on I became "Guecho," your affectionate name for me.

One evening in Puerto Rico when the folks were away, and it was just you and me at home, you decided to have a fancy meal of chicken croquettes, using china and candlelight. We ate at 7:00 p.m., "just like the rich folks do," you said, and I felt special.

You loved your nieces and nephew, and I am so glad they got a chance to know and love you. Your generosity amazed us all. When I thanked you for the chain saw you gave us, you said, "Well, I can't take it with me."

I sought your advice on curtains for our new house and you said, "I haven't given you a housewarming gift yet, so you pick out what you want, and I'll pay for it."

When I tried to thank you and said you were such a generous guy, you said "Oh, please!"

You loved to give, and it will always be an example to me. Your gentle strength, your willingness to lend a helping hand and get the job done, your sensitivity and love of beauty are some of the qualities I admire and will remember you for. I will always love you, my special brother, David.

### *Excerpts from Fran's letter to Dave*

It's over now, Dave. All over. No more suffering. No more bread box full of pills at the breakfast table or IVs seeping into your veins all day. No more facial grimacing as you valiantly try to swallow the necessary nourishment. It's over for all of us, for we suffered with you. You touched us deeply by your ability to control the intense pain while it was destroying your very life.

But you touched us in myriads of ways. Your love for beauty inspired us to search more deeply. The last three years were especially rich for us. I am glad you came to Indiana in the pregnant spring. As it delivered its celebration of color and beauty, you received much of your strength through that osmosis of new life. It seems fitting that you came to us during nature's resurrection season and lived the summer's beauty and unpredictableness as part of your own.

Now, as the fall season begins and the leaves splash their lavish brilliance, you too have dropped to the ground and become a part of the cycle as you wait for the resurrection. "There is a time to be born, and a time to die."

You were a complex person, Dave. Deep, sensitive, caring. A man of few words and rarely an unkind one. You did not share your emotions or feelings easily.

You were searching for an answer to the confusing issues which absorbed you. "Blessed are those who hunger and thirst after righteousness" now has a deeper meaning for me.

We have so many images of you in these recent years. My image of you changed from that of a quiet person, peripheral to family activities but always involved at your speed and interest level.

My image of you gradually changed further as I saw you finding your way through serious issues which too many of us accepted too glibly. Your dad and I cherish those precious discussions.

When I asked how you could cope with knowing that you had a fatal illness because you cared deeply about others who were being rejected, you said that you needed a lot of counseling and support, but accidents happen and people die from accidents. You bore that emotional and intense pain with you all these years.

We have so many rich memories. But my favorite one is seeing you bedraggled, in your sweats, looking forlorn and entreatingly saying, "Fran, I need a hug."

There is a white rose in the frivolous but beautiful Italian vase we bought in New York. Others do not understand the emptiness of the lack of beauty in a sterile hospital. We watched you suffer. We did our own suffering. We needed a promise that there is beauty beyond pain. We found it in the vase we bought in the antique shop. Perhaps it was a frivolous purchase, but it will always be a precious testimony of God's grace amid emotional pain. We will keep a rose in it as long as we are able.

Three days ago you breathed your last, and it was over. Just you, your dad, and I alone sharing that precious moment. . . . You were right, Dave, you were dying, and we are relieved that you are no longer suffering. There is so much we don't understand. Perhaps some day we will.

But rest well, David . . . rest in sweet peace.

*Lawrence's letter to Dave, October 11, 1991*
As I sit at my desk this morning, memories and tears come in waves. They remind me of the times we used to watch the waves of the Atlantic and the Caribbean surge onto the beaches of Puerto Rico. They were powerful, rhythmic, deep—and yet ending on the beach in tiny rivulets, sculpting the sand into intricate patterns of beauty. In retrospect I see those waves as a reflection of your life.

Your deep sensitivity to the hurts of people was evident already when you were very young. As I was reading a Bible story about Jesus to you and your brothers one evening, you began to cry.

When I asked why you were crying you said, "He was such a good person and they hurt him."

You continued to cry with the mistreated throughout your life. When some others were declaring the AIDS virus to be a curse from God, you were putting your life on the line to help the hurting ones. How typical of you.

Your appreciation for the beauties of God's creation was also evident from childhood. I can still see you picking wild flowers and making beautiful bouquets for your mother. I was reminded of that the other week when we were at Baintertown Park. After we sat together by the river, you went to an area which I saw as a weed patch, and you saw as a flower garden. You picked wild flowers and other plants, then made a beautiful, professionally arranged bouquet for our house.

We were not aware of how many deep friendships you had made in New York. Calls of condolence, reports that all of your colleagues in the medical records department of the hospital stood in silence in your memory and are arranging a memorial gathering—these are reminders of your contribution to the lives of others. Doña Juana, Glenn, and Tia Nana were very special persons in your life. They, like us, will miss you very much.

On Friday we placed your body in the earth in the plot you had selected, under the tree by the river, next to "Goshen Bill," the ex-alcoholic black man who worked and ministered to persons in need in this area. If you meet Bill, you probably will find you were of kindred spirit while on your earthly pilgrimage.

Your six months with us were very special. This time will be treasured as long as I live.

Hasta luego, David.

Love, Dad

*Joe's letter to Dave.*

I remember as kids collecting the offering at church on Sunday evening, then running around town undoing all Dad's good teachings. You gave me early advice in upholding the stereotype of the preacher's kid. I will miss the good times when we got together and reminisced about all our escapades as kids in Puerto Rico.

If I could emulate in a small way your generosity, kindness, and love that you have shown me and my family, we could enrich the lives of others as you have done ours.

*Galen's letter to Dave.*

Dave, it is hard to let you go because you were gentle and courageous and caring; because you loved life and shared yours with a generosity that never wanted anything in return; because you laughed easily; because you were true to yourself; because you were young and loved all things beautiful; and because you were easy to love it is hard to let you go.

I will look for you now in the early light and in the sunset. I will listen for you in the music you loved and in laughter. I will sense you in a generous deed and the kind word.

I know I will find you often, and when I do, you will surely tell me what you have always said, "Don't worry about me, brother. Don't cry for me. I'll be okay."

You left us with a lasting gift of courage, generosity, and love. We will all miss you.

◇ ◇ ◇

Pastor Waltner helped us heal by speaking of the attributes of the sun and comparing them with the attributes of God. A memorial service is an occasion for the supportive community to help heal the wound and make the remaining scar less obvious.

With the final benediction and the postlude, we were surrounded by love and undergirded by its healing strength.

Grieving is reality, but healthy grieving is done in community. Through the presence of others, we were strengthened. So many people were there to touch us, to warm us with tender kisses and empowering hugs. David's struggle was over, and they were embracing us for the lonely struggle each of us needed to bear alone.

Friends we did not expect to see blessed us with their coming. Later we learned that they too had been suffering through the journey of a gay son. Such contacts opened many doors of supportive care to those now suffering. David's sensitivity continues to bring healing to others.

The sun was now shining on someone else's dawn. After this darkness, the sun would again appear. We would continue to be warmed by the graciousness of God's love through messages, prayers, and the myriads of friends who had come to help us celebrate David's life and death.

Now it was time to honor David's request—that we have a meal together. In that teary celebrative event, as we related with our friends amid flowers, touch, and food—the basis of a wholesome life—we knew the dawn would come.

# Appendix 1 Caring for a PWA

Anyone who cares for a person with AIDS learns lessons from the experience. In the hope that it may be helpful to caregivers setting out on their painful journey alongside someone with AIDS, I want to share some of what we learned from caring for David. I will begin with specific advice, then move to more general learnings.

## Caring for David

Caring is more than making meals, doing laundry, emptying wastebaskets, picking up medications at the pharmacy, and being a chauffeur. Caring is the creative tension between doing all you know and wondering what was left undone.

- Caring is the three of us going for rides in the firefly time of evening to rejuvenate our souls and see another world not contaminated with IV poles, medications, and lung-expansion therapy.

- Caring is taking a spontaneous trip with David to a town twenty-five miles away because David decided he wanted something from a specific store.

- Caring is Rachel bringing a gallon of water with her whenever she comes because David likes the taste of that water better.

- Caring is doing your best to make a tempting, nourishing meal and watching his eyes and lips for that faint smile of approval—but not showing disappointment when he apologizes and says he can't tolerate food at this time.

- Caring is staying emotionally calm when he feels better—knowing that the moment is to be enjoyed, for it will not be permanent. A new symptom may appear tomorrow.

- Caring means wondering when the seesaw of good and bad days will end, yet not wanting to know.

- Caring means staying positive when the postman brings only bills instead of personal mail.

- Caring means having a love similar to the biblical neighbor who because of his "importunity" was granted his request. It is the incessant imploring until resistance is eroded and the wish granted.

- Caring is giving that loving hug which alleviates part of the pain's intensity.

- Caring is trying to be optimistic when he is slow, silent, and depressed—yet determined to get better, despite T cells incompatible with life.

- Caring is allowing him to write his messages when his mouth is too sore to speak or swallow, but not saying the words for him, even if it is painful to wait for his message.

- Caring is balancing your own interests with his, so his needs are not neglected and your wants not stymied.

- Caring is being there, sometimes silently—just being—and allowing the support to trickle from your heart into his.

- Caring is putting a sprig of mint in his iced tea or a rosebud on his tray, thus adding a bit of spring to his life when he is too ill to enjoy being outside.

- Caring is long rides in the unexplored community in the spring with its warming sun, threatening skies, and many promises.

- Caring is stopping silently at the roadside while he absorbs the beauty of a sunset and the aroma of new life.

- Caring is each of us worshiping the Creator in our own way.

- Caring is ordering a catered meal, using your best crystal and china, and eating by candlelight to celebrate life in the midst of the shadow of death.

- Caring is the strong arms of a father who helps his son get up from the floor after he arranged a lavish display of gladiolus.

- Caring is awakening during the night and checking on the light in his room.

- Caring is putting most of your personal plans on hold, yet being able to freely discuss needing space from each other.

- Caring is crying in the kitchen sink while alone, wondering how long one can bear to watch a loved one deteriorate.

- Caring is remembering to be grateful for the opportunity and strength to care for him. One day the lone entry in my journal was "O God, just envelop me in your love." And God did!

There is no recipe or formula for caring. When your child or equally loved one faces death from AIDS, the strength of love directs your heart. The intense love for the sufferer dare not overshadow the possibility of infection, for it is real and must be recognized.

Once the fear is understood and overcome, love will overshadow the cause of the illness, and care can be given freely and confidently. The emotions of anger, hurt, and intense sympathy will all surface at some point. There might be feelings of shame, but making judgments is in God's realm. Our responsibility is to care, regardless of the cause of the illness.

One person alone cannot adequately care for a person with AIDS. Watching someone you love being stalked by death is too stressful and consuming. Caregivers need relief and emotional release. Caring is intense, all-encompassing, and requires a diversity of abilities. Lawrence served as consultant, counselor, chauffeur, organizer, and overseer of legal matters. I was there for mothering arts. Both are needed for mutual emotional infusion.

It is not easy to face death daily or ride the seesaw of emotional highs and lows, never knowing when the formidable low will be the last. It is equally difficult to curb happiness when the sufferer is feeling better. You wish the painlessness and pleasantness could last his lifetime, but you know there will be discouragement and eventual death.

The person with AIDS (PWA) should be encouraged to be in control of his or her own life as long as possible—but boundaries must be set lest the sufferer control the caregivers. Caregivers need to accept the realities of the limitations the illness imposes, but they must find resources for their own nurturing. Brisk bicycle rides or leisurely strolls where personal agendas can be discussed are good releases.

The heaviness of the task can be lifted by joining friends for a lovely dinner along a sleepy lake, or being rejuvenated through laughter at a summer theater performance. Caring for the self is a primary requirement for caring for a PWA.

One can become so intensely involved in the life of another that there is a tendency to forget that life must be kept in perspective. It is sometimes difficult to remember that there is a world of order and laughter out there—somewhere. Maintaining contact with that world and nurturing personal relationships are necessities. One dare not allow the person's illness to rob the caregiver of his or her own emotional and physical health.

Professional and community responsibilities and involvements are important releases for personal wellbeing. During difficult times of emotional strain, personal agenda must be honored. Otherwise anger and resentment may develop. That dare not be allowed to dominate the care given.

Physical contact, a hug, or handshake is crucial to the wellbeing of any person—but especially to the one struggling to maintain life. Especially during illness we need to be touched and connected with others.

The world of touch opens the door to unspoken communication between the caregiver and the ill person. Touch is one of the most primitive sensations, and one of the first which a newborn experiences. It may also be true that it is the last the dying person perceives.

Reputable doctors and scientists stress that there is no evidence that casual contact poses a risk of infection by AIDS. However, it is wise to be tested for AIDS approximately six months after completing care for a PWA. This will relieve any anxiety the caregiver may have.

The physical care of a PWA differs only modestly from the care given to any other sufferer. The dishwasher is used more frequently. More germicides and disinfectants are used in the bathroom. Wastebaskets should be lined with plastic and emptied frequently. Caregivers need constantly to guard against any open body lesions which might come in contact with an open lesion of the PWA. They should guard as well, however, against any obvious avoidance which would make the PWA feel leprous.

Parents might initially think it cruel to allow their child to reimburse them for providing food and care, but not doing so could infringe on the independence of the PWA. If it is possible, and the PWA desires, the sufferer should be allowed to contribute to the cost of care. Developing sensitivity to the sufferer's needs is an ongoing education. There is a delicate balance between caring and caring too much.

Include generous doses of laughter in the daily care. Laughter activates release of endorphins, the body's own pain-reducing substance, and stimulates the immune system. Brighten the sickroom with cheery cards and cartoons. Tell funny stories. Develop your own sense of humor. Life for the sufferer is deadly serious. An occasional reminder that it can also be enjoyable is a pleasant and therapeutic release.

Caring for a loved one dying with AIDS can be one of the most stressful, demanding, difficult, and sad situations one can experience. But the pain is compensated by hope and faith and love which is even stronger than the emotional suffering. Caring for a dying person allows one to accept the greater gift of appreciation for the wholesome gift of life. One learns that the fear of tomorrow dare not dominate and shield one from the gift of today. Basic things previously accepted as givens—health, freedom, love, and life—become overwhelming blessings.

## Advice for Caregivers

• Except for the stigma associated with AIDS, the care of a PWA is similar to any care given to a patient facing death. Permit yourself to hate the disease but not the person with the disease. The disease deserves to be hated. The quality of care should not be affected by the diagnosis.

• Allow yourself to risk loving—even unto death, though it may feel like emotional suicide. A PWA needs the assurance that she is loved.

• Saying "I love you" implies that you will risk whatever that love implies. The word *love* is used entirely too loosely. Love is reserved for people. Be selective to whom you say those words and be prepared to pay the price. With loving comes the possibility of losing.

• Affirm the person's life. Treat the PWA as normally as possible. Let the PWA know that he is a good person loved by God. Affirm the person but not the disease.

## Advice for Visitors

• Ask the primary caregiver if the timing of a visit is appropriate. Visit as regularly as you can, and let the person depend on you. PWAs fear abandonment. If you do not come, the discouragement could be devastating. They need friends who are faithful.

• Space your visits. Allow the person to rest well and not be weakened by too many visits or visitors. The primary caregiver should schedule visits according to the patient's stamina.

• Be warm. Create a feeling of caring and warmth when you visit. Compliment the person on some aspect of his being. Build up his deteriorating self-esteem.

• Try to relax. Sometimes it takes a while to feel comfortable near PWAs. They sense that and will help you through that stage. Fear is stifling.

• Be prepared to sit through the deafening and tumultuous silence. Often suffering is too painful for words. Intellectual stimulation is sometimes too deafening. She is too weak to think. Just be there. Give the gift of silence along with the gift of presence.

• Don't expect the person to answer many questions. If he wants to talk, listen. Let the person set the tone.

• Give no advice unless asked.

• If the person desires, read an inspiring poem, or a passage from the Bible or a special book. But keep your voice clear and gently soothing. Do not read anything controversial.

• Pray if it seems appropriate. Let the PWA know that you care and are praying daily.

• Don't fuss over the person. Straightening a sheet or offering a cool hand may be soothing. But don't *insist* on doing something.

• Touching is crucially important. It is okay to hug a person with AIDS. Give some sign of affection.

• Cry with the PWA if it seems appropriate. You are both hurting, and it is all right to cry when you hurt.

• Allow your friend to express anger. If your friend is angry with you, stay calm. The PWA shows anger mainly to those with whom she feels comfortable. Don't allow yourself to become openly angry.

• Talk and listen. But most importantly, listen.

• Allow the PWA to talk about his illness. Admit that he might seem weaker and has a clear picture of his condition—but point out the unpredictability of the disease. Tomorrow might be better.

• If she talks of death, listen. Help her maintain reality and hope, but don't give hope when it is unrealistic. Do not discourage a discussion of death.

• Take your cues from your friend.

• When you are emotionally involved with a PWA, it is easy to make promises you may not be able to keep. Think seriously before you promise anything. PWAs already have more disappointments and discouragements than they can handle.

• Be consistent. If appropriate, when you leave plan the next visit, so the person has something to look forward to. Be sure to call early if you must cancel. Help your friend feel secure. Be understanding if the PWA needs to cancel because of pain.

• Let her know you are there to walk with her, but maintain your objectivity.

• Let your compassion show. Your speech will convey words. But your body language conveys the message. Convey tenderness and tolerance.

• Adapt to the situation. Humor, when appropriate, is therapeutic. Funny toys, silly artifacts, or books of humor may cause smiles.

• Flowers and food are appropriate when you know the person's allergies and dietary limits. Wilted flowers may remind the person of approaching death and should be removed.

• If you can and the person is able, plan a diversion. Take her for a short ride, for a short walk, to a movie, or wherever the friend may want to go. PWAs need change, just as you do. Provide a pleasant experience away from his regular setting.

• Unless you are a special person in the life of the PWA, make your stay short.

• Don't pretend to have all the answers. Let your humanity show. Be honest by saying you also have doubts. Identify with feelings, but never say, "I know just how you feel." None of us can know or understand the feeling of abandonment which some PWAs feel. Even persons with the same diagnosis suffer in different ways.

- If you are a longtime friend, bring family pictures to show and talk about, but do not bore with too many details. Provide opportunity for her to talk about things beyond the sickroom.

- Send postcards or notes on attractive paper between visits, or send funny cartoons, and tell him you are looking forward to the visit.

- If the PWA is too ill to talk, sit close at eye level and hold a hand. Be there. That, after all, may be the most important thing you can do.

# Appendix 2 Uncle David

*David's nephew Aaron Greaser, a junior in high school, was asked to write on the subject of his choice for an assignment. He wrote on the subject uppermost on his mind. Here is the result.*

My uncle David was very special to me. I suppose that one of the reasons was that he was my father's twin brother. But there was more than that. The way he handled his death and his dying and also the way he lived the last part of his life and how he corrected his mistakes still amazes me.

His full name was David L. Greaser. He died on October 10, 1991, at 4:35 a.m. He died of AIDS. And, yes, my uncle was gay. But he didn't get the virus through sex. You see, he was a nurse in New York City. He volunteered for an organization that helped people with AIDS. These were mostly people who had been rejected by their families and treated with contempt by society. Nurses gave people the medication that they needed to stay alive.

My uncle had given a man an injection, and he was putting the needle back into its holder. As he was doing so, he pricked his finger. A needle prick is a very small thing. I wouldn't normally call a needle prick a cause for death. But this needle caused a mortal wound because it killed Dave. And not only did it kill Dave, but it wounded his entire family, including me.

The way my uncle looked physically changed with the different stages of his illness. At the beginning he looked like a healthy man of about 180 pounds. Before this whole thing was over, he was down to around eighty pounds.

In the beginning, he looked fairly normal. He was about six feet, two inches tall. He was slightly balding, with light brown hair. Surprisingly, he didn't look much like my dad, because they were not identical twins. I couldn't figure that out when I was little, how they were twins but looked different. About the only thing he had in common with my dad was height.

I remember going to visit him close to the time when he died. He looked almost like a completely different person. He was gaunt and skeletal. His cheeks were sunk in, and his skin was a sickly hue. On his back, his spine stood out. His arms were thin and stick-like. His breathing was ragged. He wore pancake makeup to cover the worst of his sores. I have a baseball hat of his that I got after he died. It has some of his makeup on the inside sweatband. I wear it around the house.

It was hard for my uncle to speak because of all the sores in his mouth. It was also difficult for him to eat solid food. He ate a lot of that breakfast drink stuff. During this time when I saw him, he was looking better than usual. He had gotten a fresh transfer of blood a week or so before we got there. I would have hated to see him in a worse condition. He looked like a walking corpse as it was. There is no way I can totally describe how he looked to me, or how I felt during this time. It's hard for me to bring up this much as it is.

David grew up in Aibonito, Puerto Rico, along with his three brothers and one sister. His parents were missionaries there.

So they all grew up down there, speaking Spanish. And during any given time during a visit, the conversation would switch from English to Spanish. They wouldn't even miss a beat. That could and still can be very frustrating for me, because I don't speak much Spanish. But speaking Spanish helped all of them throughout life.

Out of five children, four have done some kind of translating work, Dave included. He got a degree in interior design at a university in New York, then went back and got a nursing degree. He paid his way by doing translation work for the legal system.

All of the brothers seem to have been gifted with some kind of ability related to art. My one uncle is an artist, my father makes artwork from wood, and Dave had a fine eye for fine art. He had a great appreciation for art and bought as much of it as he could. In fact, when he knew he was going to die, he bought four pieces of very fine art, one to be given to each of his siblings. We got a driftwood sculpture of an old man. It's hanging on our wall in our living room.

Dave loved art that had beauty and feeling in it. In fact, the last trip that he ever took was to the Mennonite Relief Sale in Indiana. He spent the day watching the quilts in the quilt auction.

Dave liked beauty in art and in life as well. He made trips to Texas and into the New York mountains to look at the wildflowers while they were in bloom. He also made trips to the Caribbean and the Canary Islands, for their beauty. He would travel thousands of miles just to see nature at its best. That amazes me.

Describing Dave's religious views is not easy. One of the main reasons is that nobody really knows what they were. For several years Dave rejected religion. But at the end, just before he died in the hospital, he asked for a local pastor.

It was difficult for him to speak enough to ask for that. I don't know what they talked about before Dave finally died. I'm not sure that Dave could even talk anymore. And whatever commitment he made or did not make was between him and God.

We don't know what he decided. He might have accepted Christ, and he might not have. That was one of the things that made his death so difficult, the not knowing. It is one of my greatest wishes that he did. When I pray, I pray that I will stay with God, that I will someday have children, that the world will become better, and that my uncle did accept Christ before he died.

Dave taught me more about life and death than I can begin to explain in a simple English composition. He died because he was helping those who needed his help. He loved the unlovable. He showed me that you can correct your mistakes.

He showed me how to die. He didn't embrace it. He didn't throw away all hope of life. He kept living until he was physically and emotionally unable to take anymore. He showed me that you have to face a problem. You cannot just pretend that it isn't there. He could have done that, but he didn't. He faced the facts and took whatever came to him.

Writing this has not been easy for me. I am crying right now. I put off writing this until Monday night. I put it off for two weeks because I didn't want to face what writing this would do to me. I am sitting here thinking about all the stories he and my dad told me about Puerto Rico. I'm thinking about how he looked at the end.

I didn't cry at the funeral. But I am doing it now. I'm trying to think of some clever way of ending this, but I can't. I don't even care about my paper now.

I don't care. I just want my uncle back. I want to get to know him better, and I want to tell him that I love him. He didn't have to die. I have said before that I didn't want to wish this on anybody else, to wish that anybody else had been pricked by that needle. But right now I do wish that.

I'm not crying anymore. But whatever I said above I am going to leave there. It may not be a part of your English paper, but it is a part of how I feel. I want him back.

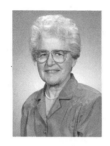

# The Author

Born in Ohio, Frances Bontrager Greaser grew up in western New York, the ninth of a family of ten children. After receiving her R.N. from Lancaster (Pa.) General Hospital, in 1950 she went to Nazareth, Ethiopia, where she worked in a rural hospital under sponsorship of Eastern Mennonite Missions for three years. On completion of her term, she and a friend spent two months traveling through Africa and Europe enroute to the United States.

In 1955 Bontrager received her B.A. in nursing from Eastern Mennonite University (Harrisonburg, Va.) and became director of nursing in a school for children with cerebral palsy near Baltimore, Maryland. Later she taught at Buffalo (N.Y.) Children's Hospital. Overseas nursing continued to appeal to her, and in 1959 she, two other nurses, and a doctor opened a rural hospital in northern Haiti under sponsorship of Mennonite Central Committee.

She received a master's degree in nursing education from Syracuse (N.Y.) University in 1962, then taught pediatrics at Goshen (Ind.) College. Later she became director of nursing in a school for the developmentally disabled in Elkhart, Indiana.

In 1975 Bontrager married Lawrence Greaser who was Latin-American director of Mennonite Board of Missions and she became a stepmother of five children and grandmother of one. The marriage did not diminish their pleasure in traveling, and together they have explored four continents. Though retired, they continue to enjoy new experiences.

Greaser is an active member of College Mennonite Church (Goshen, Ind.). In addition to exploring new places and activities, her interests include meeting and enjoying people, volunteering, entertaining, playing with and rearranging words, reading (especially biographies), creative sewing, and shopping for bargains.